Advance Praise

"Because children spend over half their time in bed, one of the most important gifts you can give them is a safe and healthy one. Bader provides credible evidence that will change how you view where your child sleeps, as well as answers for finding the safest options."

—**Janelle Sorensen**, Chief Communications Officer, Healthy Child Healthy World

"Sleep Safe reminds us of the health risks we face every day from environmental toxins and shocks us with their proximity. The chemicals found in your mattress, as with so many consumer products, are being camouflaged in greenwashing. This book will open your eyes to better choices that will steer you towards a safer, healthier lifestyle."

—**David Steinman**, author of *Safe Trip to Eden*, *Diet for a Poisoned Planet* and co-author of *The Safe Shopper's Bible: A Consumer's Guide to Nontoxic Household Products, Cosmetics, and Food*

"It was a profoundly disturbing revelation to learn about the extent of our chemical exposure during sleep as a result of outgassing from elements used in the manufacturing of mattresses and bedding. As many of us strive to make healthier, less toxic choices in our everyday lives it becomes common sense, after reading Walter's book, that one of the most important places to start the transition is in our own bedroom, where we spend up to a third of our lives sleeping. Armed with the information Walter provides, it is easy to reduce our exposure to these toxins and carcinogens by simply replacing our current choices with healthier alternatives."

—**Leanne Meyers,** Environmental Activist, CEO Prana Entertainment Group

Sleep Safe
in a
Toxic World

Your Guide to a
Safe Night's Sleep

*For Doug Parsons,
May you always Sleep Safe!
Best regards, Walt Bader*

Walter Bader

**Freedom
Press**

Copyright© 2007, 2011
First edition 2007
Second edition 2011

Disclaimer: The material in this presentation is for informational purposes only
and not intended for the treatment or diagnosis of individual disease. Please visit a
qualified medical or other health professional for specifically diagnosing any
ailments mentioned or discussed in detail in this material.

Book design by Bonnie Lambert
Cover design by Emily Kelley

ISBN: 978-1-893910-90-4
Printed in the U.S.A.

Published by Freedom Press
120 North Topanga Canyon Boulevard
Topanga, CA 90290

Bulk Orders Available: (800) 959-9797
E-mail: info@freedompressonline.com

*Dedicated to everyone striving to reduce their daily
exposures to chemicals in our increasingly toxic world.*

Acknowledgements

WHERE DOES ONE BEGIN to acknowledge all the people who have influenced our education and perspectives? If they were alive today, I would personally thank Rachel Carson, whose book *Silent Spring* first alerted me to the seriousness of air and water pollution, and people like Dr. Theron Randolph, who tried valiantly to make the public aware of the health risks associated with chemical exposures in the early 1950s. Both wrote books in 1962 that changed my life.

I would also like to thank Sylvia Seymour, whose tireless proofing was indispensable, as well as my brother, Dr. Myles Bader, who gave me encouragement and a great example to follow.

Finally, I would like to recognize the value of the thousands of consumers whose questions over the years directed me to find answers to the issues they were trying so hard to define in an effort to protect their health and the health of their families. Their questions taught me a great deal.

CONTENTS

Foreword

ONE OF THE MOST FREQUENT QUESTIONS I am asked when people consult with me about how to make their homes healthier places to live in is about bedrooms and, in particular, about beds. What is a healthy bed? Are healthy beds really that important? What's the healthiest bed? Are they worth the investment? Where do you buy one? Is organic really better? What about memory-foam beds—are they any good? That's why I am so delighted Walt Bader wrote this book. Now I can refer people to this goldmine of information that answers all these questions.

I first discovered Walt and his company, Lifekind®, several years ago on the Internet while doing research for my book, *Homes That Heal*. I was looking for the best organic bed and bedding and was really impressed with the full disclosure Lifekind gave on all their products. I remember thinking, "Finally! Someone is doing it right!" With so much "green-washing" going on today, where businesses try to make themselves look more environmentally friendly than they really are and deceive consumers with misleading claims about the all-natural wholesomeness of their products, it's increasingly difficult to find companies with vision and integrity providing genuine organic products and great customer service. Walt now brings the same vision and integrity that goes into Lifekind to this book.

The good news is that people are beginning to realize that the health of their home impacts the health of their family. Often the difference between a healthy and a toxic home is simply decided by the consumer choices we make. The bad news is that there are so many poor quality and toxic consumer products on the market, and the everyday person has no way of knowing what they are exposing themselves to. Labels and product ingredient lists rarely show all the dangerous chemicals that can go into making a product.

Thankfully, Walt decided to share his extensive research on beds and compile it into a book so it could be made available to the general public. Contained within these pages you will find a multitude of facts, scientifically valid studies and never-before-available laboratory test results revealing the chemical composition of several popular types of mattresses (such as "memory foam"). This book is essentially a full disclosure on the hidden truth about beds.

What is so important about bedrooms and beds? As Walt points out, on average we spend about a third of our life in bed. Children, the elderly and sick spend even more time there. According to the National Sleep Foundation, 50 to 70 million Americans (including children) suffer from intermittent sleep disorders, 40 million of which have chronic sleep problems. Sleep is not merely a "time out" from our busy routines; it is essential for good health, mental and emotional functioning, and safety. Sleep is when the body detoxes and heals itself. Anything that impairs our ability to sleep properly or our quality of sleep has significant impacts on the other two-thirds of our life. What most people don't realize is that the actual bed you sleep in can be the cause of many of these problems.

Sleep Safe points out that while your mattress label may tell you what your mattress is made *of*, it does not tell you what those materials are made *from*. Why would you want to know this? Because many commonly used mattress materials are a chemical nightmare. Polyurethane foam, for example, is made from a base of petrochemicals combined with a staggering array of additional chemical ingredients used as stabilizers, catalysts, surfactants, fire retardants, colorants, and blowing agents. Each of these chemicals is associated with a host of environmental problems as well as numerous human health hazards, such as chronic bronchitis, reduced lung function, breathlessness, nausea, vomiting and various allergic reactions. Some are even listed as potential carcinogens and reproductive toxins.

People also report experiencing restless sleep, frequent waking, insomnia, and waking feeling "foggy" in the morning after sleeping on certain mattresses. Though these latter effects may not be considered life-threatening, they can certainly ruin a person's productivity and quality of life. So if you are sleeping on a mattress or pillow containing materials such as polyurethane foam, you may be breathing in and absorbing through your skin these various chemicals all night, every night, as they offgas from the product. And what's more, offgassing may continue, to some degree, indefinitely for the product's entire lifetime. Why is the consumer not warned about any of this? I, for one, would want to know!

If you care about your health, it's important to learn about what you are sleeping on. Walt's lucid and comprehensive explanations will help you understand just how many layers of potentially hazardous chemicals you and your family are being exposed to each night. And it's not just your mattress. Add to the equation foundations which often contain the same chemicals as the mattress, sheets and blankets made of synthetic fibers or pesticide-laden natural fibers treated with additional chemicals for our "no-need-to-iron" convenience, and top it all off with fragranced and chemical laundry products. One can only conclude that many manufacturers have no real concern about what is in their products.

Toxic emissions from bedroom chemicals can be one of our most significant sources of daily exposure to pollution and the cause of countless maladies. Yet, when was the last time your doctor or health care professional asked you what you sleep on at night? I believe beds are one of the single-most overlooked culprits in people's (and especially children's) health problems. What if your child's frequent waking at night, inability to concentrate at school, or temper tantrums are because he is sleeping on a toxic bed? What if you are needlessly medicating your child when what she really needs is a few good nights' sleep on a healthy bed?

Some people may argue that they don't experience any noticeable negative reactions to their beds. Even so, you are still being exposed, and these low-level exposures over a long period of time can wreak havoc with your health. So do make sure you give your doctor or health care professional a copy of this book next time you see them, and ask them to review this valuable information.

Mixed throughout these pages you will also find plenty of great advice, such as how to shop for an organic mattress. No one had ever explained this to me before, and it makes so much sense. By the end of this book you will have learned everything you need to know about beds to become an informed consumer. You will also know where to begin to make your bedroom a much healthier environment to sleep in. There is everything to gain and nothing to lose as you discover for yourself the many benefits of a truly great night's sleep.

Finally, on a personal note, I began switching my family over to organic beds several years ago. I was not able to do it all at once, so I did it gradually. First I changed my family's pillows to organic wool and organic cotton. Then I changed everyone's bedding over to certified organic cotton: pillowcases, sheets, duvet covers. All of this felt wonderful to do and gave me more peace of mind at night. However, the most significant difference came when we got rid of our expensive, popular brand-name mattress and replaced it with a true organic one. That first night's sleep was blissful and I have not looked back since.

May you and your loved ones enjoy great health, wonderful sleep, and all the benefits this book offers.

—Athena Thompson
Building Biologist
Author of *Homes That Heal*

Preface

IF YOU WANT TO SEE ME SNEEZE, just give me a peppermint. As a young boy, some of my food allergies seemed funny. But it became less of a laughing matter as I got older and my allergies continued to worsen. By the time I was seven or eight, I could not walk down the laundry products aisle in the supermarket without my eyes tearing and burning. I was never too excited when my parents took me into the large toy store in town because it smelled horrible and made me feel dizzy.

Not everyone took my complaints seriously. After all, the first book about individuals with reactions to the chemicals in their environment wasn't even written until I was in college (Dr. Theron Randolph, *Human Ecology and Susceptibility to the Chemical Environment*, 1962). Like many of my generation, I was raised at a time when TV commercials promoted "Better Living Through Chemistry." DDT was sprayed throughout my local neighborhood to control mosquito populations, and great new products were being introduced made out of a wonder chemical product called "plastic." Basically, I survived my youth by submitting to countless scratch tests and injections to desensitize my allergies, and avoiding all the products and places that I realized were not for me. Still, most of the time my best friend was the biggest box of Kleenex I could find.

Today my condition would be diagnosed as Multiple Chemical Sensitivity (MCS). While for years people looked askance at this diagnosis, MCS is now recognized by reputable organizations such as The American Medical Association, The American Academy of Environmental Medicine, The National Academy of Sciences/National Research Council, The American Public Health Association, The American College of Physicians, and many more, including 22 U.S. federal entities; local, state and federal courts; and numerous international groups.

I realize today there is no way I can avoid all of the chemicals that surround me on a daily basis. But I try. My home is as chemical-free as possible, I drive a car with a good air filter, my work environment has non-VOC paint on the walls, and I sit at a non-outgassing metal desk. I even cultivate an organic garden and an organic orchard to help me avoid every chemical I possibly can.

In 1994, I decided that people might benefit from what I had learned about chemicals and the products I had incorporated into my daily lifestyle. In my desire to find a way to make this information and the products I was using available to people who were suffering from chemical sensitivities, as well as those who simply wanted to be proactive and avoid exposure to toxins in their life before it turned into a health concern, I started a national catalog company.

The company, Lifekind®, Inc., grew faster than I ever imagined, and became a portal for those who wish to research chemicals, review our Hazardous Ingredients Glossary or select a book from a list of suggested reading. Lifekind's mission is still the same: to promote products that lower your daily exposure to dangerous chemical ingredients, and to help you identify product ingredients that are potential health risks to you, your family and our planet.

I have personally believed for years that the information in this book should be made available to the public who, for the most part, are still under the illusion that government agencies are protecting their health, and that product labels give them accurate insights into a product's health risks.

This book is the culmination of my experiences, conversations with thousands of consumers, and primary research. The information has changed my life, and I promise it will change yours as well. Avoiding environmental contaminants in your mattress and bedroom is not that difficult. Incorporate these suggestions into your lifestyle, and the peace of mind alone will help you to sleep better.

Introduction

ONE OF THE MOST SIGNIFICANT CHANGES we can make to reduce our exposure to toxins and improve our overall health is to make modifications in the one location where we spend roughly one-third of our lives: our bedroom. A healthy sleeping environment will give your body a chance to recover from the toxins and stress that it is exposed to throughout the day. Given the fact that we have almost exclusive control over the furnishings, equipment, and attire we place in and near our bedrooms, it is up to us to safeguard our health by making this room as healthy and environmentally safe as possible. This book will give you the information you need to improve the health and safety of your bedroom.

Our bodies are under constant attack throughout the day from germs, toxins, pollutants, and other harmful substances. While we may try our best to minimize exposure to these pollutants, it is a daunting challenge. And the question remains…how great an assault can our bodies take from the vile concoctions mixed in with our food, cosmetics, work environment, and household products, before they collapse? This is a question that no one can answer precisely, but it stands to reason that the human immune system has its limits.

While it may come as no surprise that pollution is ubiquitous with far-reaching health consequences, many Americans would be shocked to realize that toxic emissions from bedroom chemicals may be one of our most significant sources of daily exposure to pollution. Bedroom pollutants have multiple origins, including chemicals, pest infestation, and electromagnetic fields (EMFs). Whether your bedroom is a simply furnished room or an elaborate designer masterpiece, it can be laden with chemicals that emanate from paints, varnishes, carpeting, furniture, dry-cleaned clothing, cleaners (including furniture polishes), books, magazines, window treatments, televisions and stereo equipment, and bathroom chemicals (especially plug-in air fresheners). And perhaps one of the greatest offenders is the one item in our bedroom with which we are intimately familiar: our mattress.

Each night, we approach our mattress with minimal clothing and lay down for a seemingly restful and restorative night's sleep. But in reality, while resting on a conventional mattress we are breathing in and absorbing through our skin a slew of chemicals from the synthetic fibers in paddings, pillows, fillings, bed linens, and chemical treatments—chemicals that can disrupt our sleep patterns and negatively affect our health.

Our mattresses emit gases from the toxic soup of components and applications used to create them. From the polyurethane foam used in the padding to fire retardants and antimicrobial additives, conventional mattresses can continue to release these dangerous gases long after their production. Even after the mattress has completed outgassing (if this ever occurs), its synthetic and chemically based construction provides a hospitable environment for dust and dust mites, whose excrement is the number-one trigger for asthmatic attacks.

What's worse, chemical exposure from conventional mattresses includes chemical additives you will not find disclosed on law labels (those white labels that say, "Do Not Remove"). These include polyester-cotton blends used for "ticking," vinyl for water resistance (used on both hospital and children's bedding), Dacron polyester for batting, and polyurethane foam (made from polyols and TDI, or toluene diisocyanate).

The next time you shop for a mattress, check with the salesperson for a disclosure sheet that itemizes the ingredients and lists the potential health hazards of the product. No such information is available, and the absence of this information at the time of purchase prevents you, as a consumer, from making an informed decision about the product you are contemplating purchasing. If an information sheet were available, it would inform you that TDI, a likely component of your new mattress, is recognized as a human carcinogen, and that exposure to this chemical can cause a number of health conditions, including respiratory problems such as bronchitis and asthma. Furthermore, liver damage, blood disorders, and breathing problems have been linked with vinyl chloride monomers, another known human carcinogen. Boric acid is a multipurpose roach powder that is commonly used as a fire retardant on mattresses. Yet chronic exposure to this chemical has been associated with reproductive, liver, and kidney problems. Unfortunately, it is highly unlikely that you would ever be given such information from a mattress manufacturer or salesperson.

In addition to the chemicals emitting from our mattresses, we increase our chemical exposure further by wrapping ourselves in sheets and blankets made from synthetic fibers or pesticide-laden natural fibers that are soaked in chemicals. While wrinkle-free bedding may sound good on a package label, the price we pay is exposure to unnecessary and increasing levels of dangerous chemicals, such as the widely recognized carcinogen formaldehyde.

Since our skin is our largest organ and the most porous entry point into our bodies, it is important to remember that what goes onto the skin will also go *through* the skin. It is often said that what touches our skin ends up in our cells—a frightening adage to consider the next time you are pondering a purchase of bedding, clothing, or cosmetics. Without realizing it, we may make hundreds of decisions each day that place convenience over health.

For instance, poly-fill pillows are economical, but are they worth the price the body must pay? They may be inexpensive and "hypoallergenic," but these pillows are made of synthetic chemical fibers, foam, or feathers that have been disinfected with undisclosed chemicals. These components may be a source of chemical contaminants, as well as allergens, when inhaled and absorbed into the body through the skin and lungs.

Hypoallergenic

Hypoallergenic is a word that was created by a small cosmetic company in the early 1960s, and was quickly adopted by the advertising industry to describe products that produce fewer allergic reactions.

The Greek prefix *hypo* literally means "less" or "below," so when a product is designated as hypoallergenic it means that it will conceivably trigger fewer allergic reactions in people who suffer from allergies.

The term does not relate to chemical exposures. The expression has no medical definition, and there is no certification process or organization that reviews whether a product using the word "hypoallergenic" can prove any lessening of allergic reactions.

The cumulative effects of these chemical exposures may express themselves in a number of ways, from poor quality of sleep to allergic reactions, to even more critical health concerns, such as respiratory distress and a host of other serious and life-threatening illnesses. Doctors and health experts agree that sleep is critical to improving and even maintaining our health. But many of today's mattresses, while comfortable, do little to promote our health. In fact, I believe most conventional mattresses are actually harmful to our health.

And let's not minimize the effect these chemicals can have on our children. Many children are exposed to these chemicals from the moment of conception. Throughout their development, growing babies are exposed to these chemicals in the womb, through their mother's breast milk, and then through their own chemically laden crib mattresses. Numerous studies have identified the potential reproductive and developmental health risks associated with chemical exposure. The cumulative impact of the myriad chemicals we are exposed to on a long-term basis is an issue that may continue to plague us through the years, and has the potential to significantly decrease our health over time.

Whether your interest is environmental or health-oriented, it is worthwhile to bear in mind that the effects of just one chemical or pollutant are unlikely to cause major health problems over time. Rather, it is the sum total that ultimately affects and influences long-term health. Simple changes that help you avoid chemical exposure can do wonders for building a healthier system, both human and environmental.

PART 1

The Toxic Soup: Chemicals and Your Health

YOU MAY THINK you are leading a relatively healthy lifestyle. You eat right, you exercise, you steer clear of cigarettes…so is it really possible that your body is laden with chemicals? Unfortunately, the answer is a resounding YES! Toxic chemicals are now endemic to our environment. They enter our bodies through the items we touch, the foods we consume, and in large part, from the air we breathe.

There are currently over 100,000 chemicals in use in today's modern society, of which only a small percentage has ever been tested for human health effects. Every day you are exposed to such a wide array of chemicals that it would be impossible to keep track of them all. Yet many of these toxins can have a serious impact on health and quality of life.

Most people are surprised to learn that their mattress may be one of their most significant daily sources of chemical exposure. Not only does a conventional mattress contain an amalgamation of undisclosed chemicals, but it is also the one item in our lives with which we have the most daily contact. It's time you learned what you are sleeping on.

Chapter One

The Body Burden and
the Burden of Proof

"In sleep we are all equal." —Spanish Proverb

W HAT'S MORE DISTURBING: the fact that we as a society are regularly exposed to a slew of toxic chemicals and pollutants, or that we have grown accustomed to this macabre fact? All of us carry in our bodies our own personal cocktail of toxic chemicals, as evidenced by samples of human blood, breath, hair, tissue, and body fluids. While we may like to think that someone is keeping an eye on the levels and types of chemicals entering our bodies, the sad truth is that most of our exposure to these chemicals is not from sources traditionally regulated by government agencies, such as waste sites and factories. Rather, our primary sources of chemical exposure are closer to home: from the activities, products, and materials that we allow to enter our indoor environment.

Many of us are exposed on a daily basis to a veritable laundry list of chemicals, from toxic mercury to pesticides to potentially cancer-causing by-products of plastic. These chemicals are found in measurable amounts in our blood, hair, and urine. Toxic chemicals are everywhere, present throughout our environment.

The production of synthetic organic chemicals has exploded since World War II. There are now an estimated 800,000 different synthetic chemicals in use, according to a recent press release from Senator Frank Lautenberg, chair of the Subcommittee on Superfund, Toxics and Environmental Health. To date, roughly 200 of these chemicals have been tested, and the health and environmental effects of many of these substances remain largely untested and unknown.

We all want our homes to be clean, safe places to live—a refuge from the chaos and cares of the outside world—but toxic invaders may lurk inside your home, putting you and your family at risk. Due to increased public awareness and concern about such toxic chemicals, many government and private agencies have started programs to monitor to what degree chemicals are being stored in our bodies, and what potential harm they might be doing to our health.

In the 1980s and 1990s, the U.S. Environmental Protection Agency (EPA) and other researchers conducted what was at that time a landmark study that measured personal exposure to pollutants. The study was called TEAM (Total Exposure Assessment Methodology), and its purpose was to measure personal exposure to pollutants. TEAM monitored more than 3,000 people in 18 different U.S. cities, and one Canadian province, for exposure to volatile organic compounds (VOCs), pesticides, carbon monoxide, particles, phthalates, polycyclic aromatic compounds, and other pollutants. Participants carried around personal exposure monitors that indicated what, how much, and where pollutants were affecting them. In addition, the researchers analyzed participants' breath to measure levels of both VOCs and carbon monoxide.

These studies produced an unexpected finding: Most of our exposure to pollutants occurs indoors, from products we choose to use. The consensus of each of these groups was that the risk from indoor air pollution and consumer products was far greater than most other risk factors surveyed, including hazardous-waste sites and industrial sources of outdoor air pollution.

In 2001, Bill Moyers aired a show entitled "Trade Secrets" on PBS. The show focused on the growing awareness and concern about chemicals used by industry to grow crops and make consumer products, and discussed to what extent our bodies are absorbing these chemicals. The show's title relates to the fact that the health effects of thousands of chemicals are never disclosed to consumers or governmental agencies such as the EPA because of businesses' claims that it is confidential business information or "trade secrets."

For the show, Bill Moyers agreed to be a participant at the Mount Sinai School of Medicine in New York as they studied the question of pollutant loads in the human body. Before participating, Moyers asked Dr. Michael McCally, vice-chairman of Preventive Medicine at Mount Sinai, whether he really thought they would find chemicals in his body. Dr. McCally's response was, "Oh yes ... no question. No question." The study analyzed Mr. Moyers's blood and urine. (A complete list of the chemicals found in his body can be viewed at http://www.pbs.org/tradesecrets/problem/popup_bb_02.html.)

The report indicated Moyers's blood and urine contained 48 compounds that can cause cancer in animals and are suspected or known to cause cancer in humans; 52 chemicals that have been linked to reproductive and child developmental damage; 17 chemicals that have been associated with heart damage; 21 chemicals that are known to interact with the endocrine system and lead to hormone disruption, which in turn may cause a host of diseases, including diabetes; 23 chemicals that can be responsible for damage to the gastrointestinal tract, stomach, liver, and gallbladder; 17 chemicals that are potentially toxic to the immune system; 16 chemicals that could be toxic to urinary systems, including the kidneys (which in turn play a critical role in regulating blood pressure); 25 chemicals that can have detrimental effects on the nervous system, causing symptoms such as muscle weakness, tremors, dizziness, confusion, memory loss and cognitive deficiencies; 20 chemicals that may affect reproductive fertility and pregnancies; 21 chemicals that can affect skin and sense organs, causing symptoms such as rash, itching, poor vision, and hearing, and that can even impact a person's sense of smell and taste.

Needless to say, Mr. Moyers was shocked by these findings. (Wouldn't you be?) If you're like me, you are probably left wondering if we are all carrying similar levels of chemical contamination, or "body burden." More importantly, in what ways are these chemicals impacting our health?

Since 2001, the Centers for Disease Control's (CDC) Environmental Health Laboratory, part of the National Center for Environmental Health, has published a bi-yearly report on chemical exposure in the United States, aptly named the National Exposure Report (NER). Studies done by the National Health and Nutrition Examination Survey (NHANES) that took place in 2003 and 2004 were used for the most recent report. The survey consisted of 2,400 volunteer test subjects of varying age, race and social roles. Using biomonitering techniques, the NHANES tested for 212 chemicals in the blood and urine of volunteers. 75 of those chemicals were added for testing in the most recent edition of the report. The chemicals discussed in the NER include environmental phenols, polybrominated diphenyl ethers (PBDEs), volatile organic compounds, and perfluorinated chemicals, among others, which will be discussed in more detail later in this book. A full list of the chemicals that were included in the biomonitering program can be down-loaded at http://www.cdc.gov/exposurereport/pdf/NER_Chemical_List.pdf.

Notable findings in the report include the presence of PBDEs in almost every single test subject. PBDEs were, until recently, commonly used as flame retardants in mattresses, bedding, and children's pajamas. In animal studies, PBDEs have been shown to interfere with neurological development and thyroid function, along with being linked to a host of other health issues. They were banned in California in 2004 due to the fact that they are known to accumulate in the environment and human fatty tissue, although the ban didn't take effect until 2008. Several other states have banned PBDEs, including Maine, Hawaii, New York, and Washington, D.C. Two common fire-retardant chemicals being used as replacements for PBDEs are tetrabromobisphenol-A (TBBPA) and hexabromocyclododecane (HBCD), both of which come with a host of suspicions about their environmental and health safety, and neither of which are included for analysis in the NHANES or NER.

The National Exposure Report has helped scientists, physicians, relevant government agencies, and private citizens better understand and diagnose health issues caused by exposure to chemicals. It is rather overwhelming to know, however, that over 80,000 chemicals are commonly used in American industry today, and have the potential to enter and be stored in our bodies, and I have little doubt that they are not beneficial to our health. This means that, even with the most recent 75 chemical additions, less than 3/10 of 1 percent of chemicals in use today have been tracked by the CDC using these biomonitoring techniques to see if they are being absorbed from the surrounding environment and consequentially stored in our bodies. Attempting to detect and study the effects of every chemical in use today would be impractical at best. In addition, new chemicals are being created and used at an increasingly rapid rate, and many of the new chemicals used in modern industry go untested for human health and environmental impacts.

Several additional studies have been conducted to evaluate the chemical load present in each of us. Recently, in 2006, the Washington Toxics Coalition, together with the Toxic-Free Legacy Coalition, tested the blood, hair, and urine of 10 volunteers for 6 different groups of chemicals commonly found in consumer products. Specifically, they tested for flame retardants found in mattresses and upholstered furniture, pesticides, phthalates found in toys and personal-care products, lead, mercury, arsenic, and chemicals related to Teflon frequently used in food packaging and stain-protection treatments.

Occupations and demographics of the 10 volunteers varied greatly, and included two Washington state senators, the cofounder of Earth Day, office workers, a member of the Spokane Indian tribe, a cancer survivor, and a priest. Some ate organic food, and some did not. While the test subjects certainly were varied, the results were remarkably similar.

All of the participants tested positive for a toxic soup of chemicals in their bodies. Each of the participants had from 26 to 39 chemicals inside them. All participants had some level of toxic flame retardants, phthalates, and Teflon-related chemicals in their systems. These chemicals are associated with a number of health conditions, including infertility, cancer, and learning disabilities.

While it is encouraging that the CDC and other notable agencies have taken notice and taken charge of acquiring data to better understand the effects of chemical exposure, there is a disturbing undertone to the studies. The NER website (http://www.cdc.gov/exposurereport) clearly states that the purpose of these tests is to provide data in an attempt to better understand what levels of different chemicals will cause health problems when absorbed into our bodies. This essentially makes us human science experiments.

In response to public demand and obvious health and environmental issues, the California state government has begun implementing the California Green Chemistry Initiative (CGCI), which is attempting to overhaul the way chemicals are made and used in the state of California. With time and awareness, hopefully other state and national governments will follow suit and update their, for the most part, outdated and insufficient environmental and health laws to include more strict regulations on chemical production and use.

Proposals set forth in the act include a website database (CGCI Final Report; pg 25, paragraph 2), as well as a public clearinghouse (pg 27, paragraph 2), that will disclose all "non-confidential" ingredients in products manufactured and/or sold in California and their potential environmental and health hazards. All producers at every stage of production will be required to disclose non-secretive ingredients for use by the manufacturers, retailers, and consumers that will use the product down the line. Hopefully, this will add a significant amount of transparency in products produced and used in California.

While this piece of legislation will provide consumers with far more information regarding the raw materials and processes used to make their products, it has its flaws. For example, confidential ingredients in certain products will be able to be accessed only by approved federal and state employees (pg. 25, paragraph 2). This means that companies with "secret ingredients" in their products (such as the patented and proprietary chemical makeup of a number of memory foam and blended polyurethane mattresses) will probably not be made available to the public. As of right now, California is the only state or federal government with plans to create such a portal to disclose ingredients in products (pg. 26, paragraph 5), and they are getting significant push back from manufacturers.

To truly protect Americans, chemical manufacturers should be required to perform long-term tests and have an affirmative duty to establish, in the same way the Food and Drug Administration (FDA) requires testing on new perscription drugs, that their products are safe for humans and the environment.

A new bill, AB 289, that was put into place in California in 2006 includes an addition to the Health and Safety Code (Chapter 699, Sections 57018-57020) that allows the Department of Toxic Substances Control (DTSC) to request that chemical manufacturers turn over relevant information regarding the procedures used to analyze chemicals for safety, as well as the intended use and mode of transportation for those chemicals. Companies to whom the request was sent will have one year to assemble and turn over the necessary information. In addition, manufacturers are required under this bill to notify the EPA at least 90 days in advance before they manufacture a new chemical. Like the CGCI, the new bill applies to any businesses that manufacture or sell chemicals in the state of California. The chemicals that are chosen for companies to provide information on will be made public on the DTSC and Cal/EPA websites. Any information found on those chemicals through public sources will be made available on the site as well. Unfortunately, and also similar to the CGCI, chemicals or mixtures that a company considers a "trade secret" will be reviewed and, if found appropriate, will not be released to the public.

Further information on both the CGCI and AB 289 is available on the California Department of Toxic Substances Control website, www.dtsc.ca.gov.

The CGCI and AB 289 are two giant steps forward in resolving the health and environmental issues put forth when common products are made and used. The goals set forth in the initiative are ambitious and complex, however, and will require extensive time and funding. Significant effort and cooperation will need to be put forth from government agencies, businesses, and private citizens in order for the proposed changes to take place and the legislation to be effective. The best strategy as individual consumers is keeping all products we consume as safe as possible instead of waiting for legislation to tell companies which chemicals they can and can't use. Simply eliminating as many chemicals as possible in our everyday lives is the most effective way to ensure the health and safety of ourselves and our families. An organic bedroom is the very best place to start eliminating chemicals due to the amount of time we spend there, and the sheer amount of chemicals we may be exposed to in that long-term breathing environment. This is not to mention the close contact our bedding has with our skin, which is the largest organ and the most susceptible way for chemicals to enter our bodies.

Hopefully, these pieces of state legislation will help to set national examples and encourage the short- and long-range studies necessary to evaluate the low-level, chronic chemical exposures that we all face on a daily basis.

On July 22, 2010, the Committee on Energy and Commerce, headed by House Representative Henry A. Waxman, introduced the Toxic Chemicals Safety Act (H.R. 5820), which aims to update the antiquated Toxic Substances Control Act of 1976. The original Toxic Substances Control Act exempted the chemical manufacturers from providing any safety information to the EPA for all chemicals produced before 1979, and the chemical industry is not about to voluntarily pursue research or publish information that could create legal liabilities. The EPA has proved ineffectual at evaluating the safety and healthfulness of chemical exposure, and even if they had been funded and staffed for the task, corporate claims of proprietary formulas (trade secrets) and confidential business information often block their inquiries.

In a testimony regarding the necessity of H.R. 5820, Ken Cook, head of the Environmental Working Group (www.ewg.org), stated that "Because the Toxic Substances Control Act of 1976 leaves the government so stunningly powerless to deal with the toxic soup from chemicals in the environment and, indeed, in the blood of all of us, the American people have lost confidence, have lost trust, that the products they are using, the chemicals they are being exposed to, are safe." A written version of the oral testimony can be downloaded from http://www.ewg.org/ken-cook-proposal-to-reform-federal-chemicals-law.

The 2010 Toxic Chemicals Safety Act gives the EPA the necessary power and funding to better monitor and control chemical production and public exposure to potentially harmful chemicals, and will expand government research and regulation of chemically produced substances. A summary of the act, as well as the entire text, can be read at http://energycommerce.house.gov.

The new act will update the original to include chemicals that weren't included before, mainly because they hadn't been invented yet or hadn't been tested for safety. A group of 19 chemicals will be included immediately, and the list is required to be expanded by the administrator to include 300 chemicals within a year of the act's implementation (section 6; pg 42, line 18). The complete list of these chemicals can be found on page 41, line 21, through page 42, line 17, of H.R. 5820. This list will be updated regularly, and will be made available to the public via a website database. Chemical manufacturers will be required to submit the chemicals and mixtures that they produce, as well as the testing methods used and deter-minations regarding environmental and health dangers, although some exceptions will be made (section 14; page 86). Like the CGCI, the Toxic Chemicals Safety Act will aim to regulate chemicals at their source rather than at their disposal. Predictably, chemical companies are not enthusiastic about the new bill.

Due to increased awareness and concern about the health problems being linked to manufactured chemicals, new laws and legislation are being put into place to give consumers more protection from unsafe and untested chemicals. Both the CGCI and the Toxic Chemicals Safety Act of 2010 are aimed at regulating chemical production and use and making information on which chemicals go into products, and their potential hazards, much more publicly available. The burden of educating ourselves and making the best choices in which products to buy and consume is still, and will remain, to be largely with us. While some of the most dangerous chemicals will be regulated more strictly, many will still be allowed in production processes. In addition, new synthetic chemicals are being produced more and more rapidly, making it impossible to test them all for environmental and human safety in a timely manner.

So how can individuals defend themselves from chemical exposures? BY AVOIDING AS MANY OF THEM AS POSSIBLE! This book will show you how.

Chapter Two

When Did Mattresses

Become So "Chemical"?

"The best bridge between despair and hope is a good night's sleep."
—E. Joseph Cossman

The Evolution of the Mattress

HISTORY HAS SHOWN time and time again that the way we choose to sleep greatly affects our quality of life. We do not sleep on mattresses by coincidence, but rather because of a basic human desire to be comfortable. Twelve thousand years ago, before humans slept on mattresses, they slept on the ground or on stone beds covered with animal skins. Mattresses only appeared around 5,000 years ago, and luxury mattresses began to appear during the early Roman era.

Through the years, humans were very creative in developing a comfortable and safe environment on which to rest their tired bodies. Beds have been made from piles of leaves; folded linens; hammocks made from straps, ropes, and webbing; woven reed mats; and rugs. They have been constructed from raised wooden boxes topped with sacks stuffed with straw, feathers, wool, horsehair, pea shucks, corn silk, coconut hair, and even seaweed. Around 3,000 BC, the first cotton mattresses were developed in Mesopotamia, Egypt, and Babylonia. The first water-filled beds were goatskins filled with water, used in Persia more than 3,600 years ago.

The bed, as a piece of furniture, was considered for many years the most important piece of furniture in the house. Many cultures have even regarded the bed as a status symbol. In ancient Egypt, beds were more than just places for sleeping—they were also places to eat meals and entertain socially.

The Age of the Roman Empire, at the turn of the first century, marked the beginning of the first luxury bed. Mattresses were stuffed with wool, feathers, reeds, or hay. They were decorated with paint, bronze, silver, jewels, and gold. During the Renaissance Period, mattresses were constructed by stuffing inexpensive fabric with the usual straw and feathers, and then placing the sack inside a more luxurious material such as silk, velvet, or satin. These mattresses were often placed on lattice-worked rope frames to elevate them so that they were not in contact with the often insect-infested floor. This practice also improved air circulation under the bed and helped to prevent mold. Today, this is one of the main functions of a mattress foundation.

Around the middle of the nineteenth century, bed frames made out of cast iron became very popular. These frames raised mattresses further from the floor and made it more difficult for insects to nest inside mattresses. (Unfortunately, since many beds during this period were commonly made from local field cotton and horsehair, the insects may well have been in the raw materials when the bed was constructed.)

Another dramatic evolution occurred during the nineteenth century with the invention of the steel-coil spring. These springs were originally invented during the Industrial Revolution, and were first patented for use in a chair seat in 1857. In 1871, a German man named Heinrich Westphal developed a mattress that utilized these springs for its supporting core.

The "modern" waterbed was introduced in 1873 by Sir James Paget at London's St. Bartholomew's Hospital. Because waterbeds allowed mattress pressure to be evenly distributed under the body, Sir Paget hoped this new style of bed could be used as a treatment for the prevention of bedsores. By 1895, waterbeds that basically looked like large hot-water bottles were being sold via mail order by the British department store, Harrods. Due to a lack of suitable materials at the time, however, the waterbed did not gain widespread use until after vinyl was invented in the twentieth century.

Modern mattresses with innerspring workings were first commercialized in the late nineteenth century, but it wasn't until the post-World War II era that chemical components were introduced into the mattress manufacturing process. Their introduction was the result of new wartime chemical discoveries, along with the need of chemical companies to find new consumer products that could utilize military technology and expanded production facilities that had been created for the war effort.

The most commonly used modern mattress material is polyurethane foam. Created in Germany in 1937, it was used extensively in mattresses as a cushioning material beginning in the 1950s, replacing natural rubber latex, primarily because of convenience and a much lower cost. Chemical giant DuPont began producing polyester fiber for mattresses and upholstered furniture in 1959. By 1965, synthetic fibers represented approximately 40 percent of all American textile-mill consumption.

The late twentieth century brought 100 percent foam-rubber mattresses, pillow-top mattresses, pocket-spring mattresses, adjustable beds, and even airbeds. The modern mattress has now become a collection of chemicals and synthetic fibers. Unfortunately, the safety of these components, both on their own and in combination with each other, may be causing significant damage to our health.

The Modern Mattress

Today's mattress may be more comfortable than its predecessors; however, this comfort has been gained at the cost of human and environmental safety. The materials used to make a modern conventional mattress may pose a serious health risk to the sleeper, and risks to our environment from the production of the components it contains, as well as the mattress's disposal in a landfill after its useful life has ended.

Take a close look at the white tag attached to your mattress—the one labeled "Do Not Remove." Mattress manufacturers are required by law to list the contents of the mattress, broken down by percentage, on this tag. This label may tell you what your mattress is made *of*, but it does not tell you what those materials are made *from*. For example, polyurethane foam is one of the most commonly used materials in modern mattresses. This material may be listed on the content label, but you will not receive any information about the potential hazards caused by the chemicals that are used to make polyurethane foam. Nor is there any information about the by-products of these chemicals, or what will happen as they break down over time.

S. Morales from Portland, Oregon, was surprised by the lack of information given to her when she purchased a new mattress a few years ago. While she was at the store, she began to feel foggy, irritable, and itchy. After sleeping on her new mattress for about three hours, she woke up with body aches and pains. She quickly concluded that the mattress was causing her symptoms. The following day, Ms. Morales's symptoms increased. "The symptoms were so unbearable that I quickly had the mattress moved and stored in a distant room in the house," she said. "My symptoms quickly vanished once I was no longer in contact with the mattress."

Ms. Morales was never informed about the chemicals or potential side effects that could be generated by exposure to her mattress. She purchased it on the assumption that it would be both safe and comfortable to sleep on. Fortunately, she was able to make the connection between her mattress and her symptoms on her own. By returning her new mattress she was able to avoid months, or possibly even years, of chronic health problems. But many people experience deteriorating health without realizing that it could be caused by their mattress. Unless they are told otherwise, they assume that their mattress and the components used to produce it are safe for their health.

In January 2002, the Boston television station WCVB-TV produced an investigative report regarding the number of consumers who had been complaining of "smelly beds." In response to this story, Foamex International, the makers of flexible polyurethane foam, issued a statement claiming that their production supply may have become contaminated with a chemical known as trichloroanisole, or TCA. Foamex International also stated that TCA poses no known health risk. However, this chemical can cause severe irritation and/or chemical burns to the eyes, skin, and mucous membranes. In addition, inhalation of TCA can result in choking, coughing, dizziness, weakness, or swelling of the throat and lungs.

According to the Consumer Product Safety Commission, tens of thousands of mattresses were recalled due to this "bad batch" of foam produced by one company and supplied to many conventional mattress manufacturers.

In order to properly evaluate the human and environmental safety of a particular mattress, we as consumers need to do a bit of research and go beyond the information that is printed on its minimally disclosing label. And the best way to do that is to become familiar with how exactly a modern mattress is constructed.

Chemical Alert…What's in Your Mattress?

- Polyurethane Foam
- Synthetic Fibers
- Volatile Organic Compounds
- Formaldehyde
- Boric Acid
- Adhesives
- Pesticides
- Herbicides
- Fungicides
- Artificial Dyes

The Mattress

Although every mattress will contain slightly different components, the modern mattress is constructed of three basic parts: the covering fabric, paddings, and a supporting core.

1. Covering Fabric: Often referred to as "ticking," the covering fabrics of traditional mattresses in years past were made from natural fibers, such as cotton, hemp, wool, or silk. Modern mattresses have replaced these natural fibers with synthetic thermoplastic fibers, such as polyester, nylon, polypropylene, acrylic, and polyvinyl chloride (PVC). Some mattresses are made from a blend of synthetic fibers and cotton. Almost all cotton used in modern mattresses, however, is grown using environmentally harmful chemical pesticides, fungicides, herbicides, and defoliants.

A mattress's covering fabric can be made of several layers, depending upon the level of insulation and support. These layers are then covered with a final quilted outer layer. This top layer is usually made of light foam or other synthetic fibers stitched to the underside of the ticking, and is the layer the sleeper first feels when lying on the mattress.

The covering fabric is subjected to a number of chemical applications such as toxic dyes, stain and water repellents, wrinkle-resistant treatments, antifungicides, pesticides, fire retardants, and antimicrobial coatings. Remember, however, that none of these chemicals are listed on the mattress law label or on any of the manufacturing literature provided to the consumer at the time of purchase.

In contrast, consider the covering fabric used in the construction of an organic mattress: certified organic cotton. Cotton that is certified organic is grown and processed without the use of any of the chemicals mentioned above.

2. Paddings: The padding layers insulate the mattress and add structure and support to its construction. These layers are most often made of polyurethane foam, convoluted foam, synthetic-fiber pads, and/or polyester fibers. In order to produce this padding, or "batting," fibers are fed into a machine in which they are combed in parallel rows and laid into a form called the "blanket."

The loft and weight of the batting is determined by the number of layers used in the blanket. At this point the blanket can be bonded or unbonded, depending upon whether chemicals are applied to it. Unbonded batting is not exposed to additional chemical treatment. It is loose in construction, and may develop high and low spots unless it is covered with cheesecloth or another lightweight fabric. Bonded batting, on the other hand, is coated with an artificial resin of acrylates in order to bind the fibers together and prevent fiber migration.

Again, compare this with the construction of an organic mattress. The padding layers are made from natural fibers such as wool and cotton, neither of which is grown or bonded with chemicals.

3. Supporting Core: Mattress supporting cores are made from latex, a variety of polyurethane formulations (including memory foam), or steel innersprings. Lately, we are also seeing the use of coconut fibers that have been rubberized or glued together into a block and used in mattress construction.

The purpose of the supporting core is to hold the body in alignment by "pushing back" in response to the sleeper's weight. This provides the mattress's overall support. In most modern mattresses (except for foam-only models), the core is made of steel coils or springs. This type of supporting core is also referred to as "innerspring." The quality of an innerspring mattress is determined by the number and type of coils that are used in its construction—basically, the more coils it has, the more support it offers.

Although the functional components of all mattresses are similar, each mattress is constructed with its own unique combination of materials. Organic mattresses use basically the same construction methods as conventional mattresses. The mattress construction materials are just different.

Most mattress manufacturers do not produce their own raw materials or components, and each vendor or supplier of raw materials may use its own combination of chemicals and manufacturing techniques. This makes it very difficult—if not impossible—for the average consumer to get a comprehensive idea of what his or her mattress is made both *of* and *from*.

The Foundation

Most mattresses are constructed to rest on another structure, known as a "foundation." They are made with the same components as a mattress, but with different construction goals. Modern mattress foundations are constructed with some combination of wood, steel springs, rigid polyurethane, high-density polypropelene, straps, covering fabrics, synthetic paddings, nails, staples, and adhesives.

There are three main types of foundations: traditional wood foundations, box springs, and grid foundations.

1. Wood Foundation: This type of foundation is usually made of fir or a similar hard wood. It typically consists of seven or eight wooden support slats that are covered with cardboard or beaverboard. This type of foundation, known in the industry as a "zero-deflection unit" or wood-slat foundation, increases a mattress's feeling of firmness or stability.

2. Box Spring: Box-spring foundations utilize extra-heavy-duty springs to give the mattress a softer or bouncier feel. If the number of springs is designed to match the mattress, it is called a "coil upon coil" box spring.

3. Grid Foundation: These utilize steel, wood, or a combination of both in a standard cross-over design to provide support for the mattress.

The labels on foundations suffer from the same scarcity of information as do those on mattresses. This denies us, as consumers, the opportunity to thoroughly evaluate the health and environmental hazards associated with these products.

Organic mattress foundations, on the other hand, offer the consumer a more healthful alternative to chemically laden foundations. An organic foundation may be either a box spring that is designed to work with an innerspring mattress, or a wood-slat foundation that is often used with a natural rubber latex mattress. Organic box-spring foundations typically contain the same heavy-duty coil springs as conventional foundations, covered with a layer of durable certified organic cotton canvas, padded with certified organic cotton batting, and then covered with certified organic cotton fabric.

Organic wood-slat foundations are generally made from cabinet-grade, untreated wood. The wood is covered with a layer of durable organic canvas, then padded with certified organic cotton batting, and finally covered with woven certified organic cotton fabric.

Natural Fibers

Cotton

Approximately 55 percent of all fibers used for clothing and home furnishings (including mattresses) in the United States are natural cotton. Used as far back as 3000 BC, it has certainly passed the test of time.

Primarily composed of cellulose (80-90 percent), cotton is usually grown with pesticides, often scoured or washed with a caustic soda, and bleached to remove the natural color. However, the certified organic cotton used in organic mattresses should not be grown with pesticides or processed with chemicals.

Since certified organic cotton is not scoured or bleached, the leaf grade, which describes the percentage of cotton-plant particles, is critical. For instance, the company I am familiar with purchases only number-one grade, which has no cottonseeds or vegetative matter to speak of after just a natural machine combing or carding. Leaf grades of commercial and certified organic cotton can be as high as grade eight. At this level, cotton looks brown rather than white and has an abundance of leaves, seeds, and twigs. I am personally familiar with organic mattresses that use this grade and boast on their labels that they are manufactured from organic cotton. Unfortunately, no state or federal labeling is required that describes the grades or processing of cotton.

Cotton is a great absorber. Accordingly, it is susceptible to pre-harvest and post-harvest contamination. Growing cotton without pesticides can be certified by independent third parties, but no procedure or sampling method exists that can assure consumers that a particular bale has not been exposed to bacteria, yeasts, molds, or other contaminants during storage, transport, or processing. Only one organic mattress company uses a non-chemical sanitization method to ensure against potential contamination.

Wool

While cotton is by far the main plant-based fiber used around the world, wool is the number-one animal fiber. Similar to cotton, wool has been around a long time. Babylonians were reputed to be wearing clothing of crude-woven wool in 4000 BC, and its attribute of being cool in summer yet warm in winter, while at the same time being fire and bacteria resistant, is a hard combination of advantages to beat.

Primarily composed of a protein called keratin, which gives it fire retardancy, wool also has a natural "crimp," or curl, that makes it resilent and resistant to crushing. Wool makes a great renewable fiber for padding mattresses.

Often I hear questions as to the origins of the wool being used in mattresses and whether the wool is taken from humanely sheared or slaughtered animals. Wool from animals killed for meat is called "pulled wool," and it represents a low-quality fiber that does not compare favorably with hand-sheared virgin wools that are not treated in any way before processing.

After shearing, wool is washed in baths containing water, soap, and soda ash. Lanolin is a byproduct of wool washing, and is subsequently recycled into a wide variety of household products. Wool used in mattresses and furniture then goes through a non-chemical process known as "carding" in which the fiber passes through a series of metal teeth that align the fibers and remove any residual organic matter. Minimally processed and locally grown, it is an excellent natural product for use in organic mattresses.

In my opinion, as a wool buyer, there are three important criteria that have to be balanced when purchasing wool. First, the chemicals that are used in the raising of the animals: sheep dips, washing formulas, and medicines administered for a variety of ailments. Second is how humanely they are treated from birth through shear. Some countries, such as Australia, are still practicing a procedure known as "mulesing," in which large areas of skin are sliced from the buttocks of lambs without anaesthetic! The reason given for this brutal treatment is that it helps prevent a painful and sometimes deadly condition known as "flystrike." After seeing this procedure in vivid living color, my stomach prevents me from buying this wool even if it has organic certification.

My third consideration is the carbon footprint of the wool. The wool I buy comes from California herds at which we have been personally present for shearing. My personal relationship with the farmer goes back years, and I am absolutely comfortable that the animals are treated humanely and the dips and washing are ecologically acceptable.

Machine-washable Wool

Almost all antifelting (getting wool not to felt or shrink) is accomplished today using what is known as the Chlorine-Hercosett process. The process removes the scales of the natural wool fibers and creates a modified smooth synthetic-type fiber by using a strongly acidic chlorine solution followed by a polymer resin.

This method has two dimensions that concern me: Individual health risks and environmental degradation. Plus, the textile industry consumes a high level of water for their various processes.

Personal Health Risks

Chlorine is recognized worldwide as a hazardous chemical, and has been linked to cancer and lung and heart disease for years. People with pre-existing lung or heart disease may be particularly sensitive to the effects of chlorine.

Usually combined with other chemicals, chlorine is used to disinfect water, purify metals, bleach wood pulp, and modify wool fiber. Exposure to chlorine gas can come in the form of outgassing from wool products that have been treated with a chlorine process.

The body absorbs chlorine gas when small amounts pass through the skin and lungs. Chlorine levels in the range of 0.01-0.019 parts per million can be discerned by most noses, but it is my opinion that risks from inhalation are still present when low-level, long-term exposures are considered.

As stated in many places within this book, my philosophy has always been to avoid as many products as possible that could pose potential chemical exposure.

Ecological Risks

Wastewater from wool plants using the Chlorine-Hercosett process to achieve machine-washable wool has high levels of absorbable organic halogen compounds (AOX). AOXes may be volatile substances like trichloromethane (chloroform), chlorophenols and chlorobenzenes, or complex organic molecules like dioxins and furans. However, most AOXes are chlorine-containing molecules, and it is generally accepted that chlorinated chemicals within the AOX family are toxic to fish and other aquatic organisms at low concentrations.

Machine-washable wool may sound great, but I have seen no consumer information that establishes that long-term exposure to these products is without risk.

Kapok

Often the tallest trees in a rainforest and now considered endangered, the 150-foot-tall kapok tree produces a fluffy cotton-like seed covering that is seven times less dense than cotton. Also known as silk cotton or Java cotton, kapok is naturally moisture-resistant, making the fiber quick-drying as well as resilient. However, it is a highly flammable product and because of its short fiber, has a tendency to crush.

Since it is grown primarily in Africa, South America, and Indonesia, kapok has a relatively high carbon footprint when compared to locally available fibers.

Coconut Coir

Looking much like a block of brown, tangled yarns glued together, this vegetative material found between the hard, internal shell and outer coat of a coconut has been used for ages to make floor mats, brushes, brooms and twine. Today, about 55 billion coconuts are produced annually and made into products, primarily in India and Sri Lanka.

The main attraction this product holds for the mattress and furniture industry is cost. Today, consumers expect to pay more for a thicker mattress, and manufacturers have to produce products that meet their expectation. As oil-derived raw materials become more scarce and expensive, manufacturers are seeking other materials to "bulk up" their constructions with lower-cost components.

While mattress cores made with coconut coir may be less expensive, they come with a significant environmental and social cost.

Quoting from an abstract done for the *International Journal of Environmental Studies*, 1997, titled "The Pollution of Retting Coconuts on the Southwest Coast of India" by S. Bijoy Nandan, "Retting activity has caused large scale organic pollution along with the mass destruction of the flora and fauna, converting sizeable sections of the backwaters into virtual cesspools of foul-smelling, stagnant waters. High values of hydrogen sulphide, ammonia, BOD_5 associated with anoxic conditions, and low community diversity of plankton, benthic fauna, fish, shell fish, wood-boring and -fouling organisms were the outstanding feature of the retting zones." In plainer language, common pollutants found in the water effluence included tannin, toxic polyphenols, pectosan, and a number of bacterial contaminants, including salmonella. In addition to the potential for water pollution, the fermentation process, inherent in the natural processing of the coir, releases methane gas, which contributes to produce a greenhouse gas that is 28 times greater than CO_2 emissions. While the crop uses few pesticides, its overall ecological footprint is concerning.

Converting the rough coir outside the inner nut into a usable commercial product frequently utilizes hand processes that take place in a variety of third-world, often poorly regulated production environments which, although in transition to more mechanical methods, still employ hundreds of thousands of workers in potentially low-level bargaining and desperate employment circumstances. Jobs range from employing people to transport, soaking and hand-beating the retted pulp with wooden mallets, and hand carding the fibers.

To date, there are no third-party certified organic coir mattress cores, although some manufacturing facilities are using a certified organic latex sap as the adhesive or bond for the fibers.

Commercially Produced Fibers

Regardless of whether fibers are natural or synthetic, their commercial production utilizes a slew of toxins and hazardous chemicals. Natural-fiber cotton is one of the worst offenders. Cotton uses approximately 25 percent of the world's insecticides and more than 10 percent of its pesticides, including herbicides and defoliants. In fact, it takes roughly one-third of a pound of chemicals to grow enough cotton for just one T-shirt.

In 2003, 84 million pounds of pesticides were sprayed on the 14.4 million acres of conventional cotton that was grown in the United States. This places cotton second (behind corn) in the total amount of pesticides sprayed, according to the U.S. Department of Agriculture. In the same year, over 2.03 billion pounds of synthetic fertilizers were applied to conventional cotton, making it the fourth most heavily fertilized crop (behind corn, winter wheat, and soybeans). The EPA considers seven of the top 15 pesticides applied to cotton in the United States in 2003 (acephate, dichloropropene, diuron, fluometuron, pendimethalin, tribufos, and trifluralin) as "possible," "likely," "probable," or "known" human carcinogens.

Table 1 lists the quantity of each of these chemicals applied to U.S. crops each year in the production of cotton.

Table 1: Carcinogenic Chemicals Used in U.S. Cotton Farming

Carcinogenic Chemical	Pounds of Chemical Applied Per Acre to Crop Each Year	Total Applied (Pounds)
Acephate	1.00	2,537,000
Dichloropropene	0.77	378,000
Diuron	0.49	1,738,000
Fluometuron	0.77	755,000
Pendimethalin	0.73	1,813,000
Tribufos	0.63	2,383,000
Trifluralin	0.83	4,156,000

Source: Adapted from U.S. Department of Agriculture, "Agricultural Chemical Usage 2003 Field Crops Summary," National Agricultural Statistics Service Ag Ch1 (04)a, May, 2004.

Synthetic Fibers

Synthetic fibers such as polyester are also commonly used in the production of mattresses. Polyester was first introduced in the 1950s, replacing rayon and nylon in many fabrics and further reducing the percentage of textiles made from cotton. Some polyesters contain chlorine, and these have become sources of harm to wildlife and humans during their production and use, as well as in the disposal of the end product.

Health experts are also beginning to uncover the connection between synthetic bedding and the development of respiratory problems such as asthma. In a study conducted at Australian National University in Canberra, researchers investigated the role of synthetic bedding materials in the development of childhood wheezing. The study involved 863 children who participated in an infant survey in 1988 and an asthma study in 1995. About 64 percent of children were exposed to a single synthetic material, 27 percent used natural-fiber bedding, and the remainder were exposed to composite synthetic bedding. By the age of seven, the children who had been exposed to composite bedding were more than twice as likely to have recently experienced night wheezing compared with children who used natural bedding. The results of the study showed that bedding exposures in infancy are prospectively associated with the development of childhood wheezing.

Polyurethane Foam

Polyurethane, first produced in 1937 by a German scientist named Otto Bayer, was created as a substitute for natural rubber. Although flexible polyurethane foam can be produced with many different chemical formulations and in several densities, in general it is made from three main raw ingredients: crude oil, natural gas, and sodium chloride.

Although you may see "polyurethane foam" listed as a component on your mattress label, the truth is that there is no one standard formula or specification for its manufacture. All flexible polyurethane foam is created in either a mold or slab process by combining chemicals known as isocyanates and polyols with other chemicals that act as stabilizers, catalysts, surfactants, fire retardants, colorants, and blowing agents. Each of these chemicals is associated with a host of environmental and human health hazards.

Isocyanates

Isocyanates are highly reactive chemicals, and there are several types that can be used to produce polyurethane foam. These chemicals are very irritating to human tissue, namely the mucous membranes of the eyes and the respiratory tract. Direct contact with liquid isocyanate can cause swelling and reddening of the skin and severe eye irritation. According to a technical bulletin produced by the Alliance for the Polyurethanes Industry, "Individuals also may become sensitized to diisocyanates and experience severe asthma-like attacks whenever they are subsequently exposed to even minute amounts of diisocyanate vapor."

Toluene diisocyanate is the most widely used starting material for polyurethane. It is made from chlorine, toluene, phosgene, sulfuric acid, and nitric acid, all of which are considered hazardous volatile organic compounds (VOCs). Toluene diisocyanate is associated with a number of health hazards, such as pulmonary injury, chronic bronchitis, reduced lung function, breathlessness, immunologic lung disease, nausea, vomiting, and allergic reactions. Allergic and immune-system responses occur when this chemical reacts with molecules in human tissue and/or blood to form a new compound. This new compound then triggers a negative reaction within the body. In addition, toluene diisocyanate is listed as a potential carcinogen by the National Toxicology Program and the International Agency for Research on Cancer. Approximately 31,000 pounds of toluene diisocyanate are produced by 23 polyurethane foam manufacturers in 100 plants throughout the United States every year.

In recent years, another isocyanate—known as 4-methylenediphenyl diisocyanate—has become popular in the production of polyurethane foam. This chemical is made from formaldehyde, sulfuric acid, nitric acid, phosgene, and benzene. According to the EPA, short-term inhalation of high concentrations of this chemical may cause sensitization and asthma in humans. Contact with the skin has been known to induce dermatitis and eczema in those who work in foam-production facilities. It is also known to irritate the skin and the eyes of rabbits. Over the long term, inhalation of 4-methylenediphenyl diisocyanate has been shown to cause asthma, dyspnea, and other respiratory impairments in workers.

Polyols

When polyurethane foam was first produced, it was made using polyester polyol. Today, the polyol most commonly used is a polyether polyol, based on the use of alkylene oxides such as ethylene and propylene oxides. These chemicals are produced from the cracking and distillation of petroleum.

Additives

Other chemicals used to produce polyurethane foam include surfactants, catalysts, fire retardants, dyes, and blowing agents. At one time, chlorofluorocarbons were used to produce the softer, lower-density foams, but these chemicals have since been banned due to their ozone-depleting characteristics. The industry has moved towards methylene chloride, a chemical that is listed by the EPA as a probable human carcinogen that is also associated with damage to the nervous system and decreased visual and auditory acuity. The production of polyurethane foam releases approximately 24 million pounds of this chemical into the atmosphere in the U.S. each year. In fact, according to a report produced by the National Resources Defense Council and the World Resources Institute, methylene chloride produces the largest release of any carcinogen into the air in the United States.

"Green" Polyurethane Foam

There has been a surge of polyurethane mattresses and bedding products that are now calling themselves "green" (or some shade of green).

As previously mentioned, many of the chemicals used to make polyurethane are recognized carcinogens, and some of the fire retardants used in the foam formulas increase a mattresses's chemical toxicity. And don't forget that polyurethane does not decompose in landfills and increases our dependency on oil, which is the main base material.

What is being touted today as a "green" polyurethane mattress claims to be natural, organic, eco-friendly, and sustainable because the manufacturer has altered its formulas with a soybean, castor bean, or other plant-derived polyol. The consumer will see an advertisement or promotion saying that this mattress is made with 20 percent or some other percentage of soy, and that percentage makes the product "green," "greener," or "greenest."

Earlier I pointed out that polyurethane is primarily composed of approximately equal parts isocynate (the gas that killed thousands in Bhopal, India) and a polyol. So if you substitute a soy-based polyol for 20 percent of the 50 percent, you would have a product that is 10 percent soy and 90 percent disastrous chemicals. Even if all the traditional polyols were replaced with soy-based polyol, the product would still be made up of 50 percent isocynate. Hardly green, or perhaps we could call it "slightly green."

A few other concerns I have regarding soybeans revolve around whether or not they are genetically modified (GMO) crops, which describes over 90 percent of the soybeans grown in the United States according the U.S. Department of Agriculture. This is also the crop that is a favorite for planting on the "reclaimed" Amazon rainforests. It is a valuable source of food that could be used to feed people instead of being used in industrial applications.

Altering traditional polyurethane formulas by adding natural and synthetic latex has also become a popular way to claim a greener heritage. Although the formula variations are endless, if the end product is called polyurethane its basic characteristics are still the same.

Flammability

Polyurethane foam is also highly flammable, and is often referred to by fire marshals as "solid gasoline." Therefore, flame-retardant chemicals must be added to its production when it is used in mattresses and upholstered furniture. This application of chemicals does not alleviate all concerns associated with its flammability, since polyurethane foam can release a number of toxic substances at different temperature stages. For example, at temperatures of about 800°C, polyurethane foam begins to rapidly decompose, releasing gases and compounds such as hydrogen cyanide, carbon monoxide, acetonitrile, acrylonitrile, pyridine, ethylene, ethane, propane, butadiene, propionitrile, acetaldehyde, methylacrylonitrile, benzene, pyrrole, toluene, methyl pyridine, methyl cyanobenzene, naphthalene, quinoline, indene, and carbon dioxide.

Of these chemicals, carbon monoxide and hydrogen cyanide are considered lethal. Carbon monoxide is a colorless, odorless gas that cannot be detected by the human senses. When breathed in, it deprives the body of oxygen, resulting in dizziness, headaches, weakness of the limbs, tightness in the chest, mental dullness, and finally a lapse of consciousness that leads to death.

Hydrogen cyanide is a colorless gas that carries the odor of bitter almonds. This gas paralyzes the respiratory center of the brain, causing dizziness, headaches, shortness of breath, convulsions, and coma. In high concentrations, inhalation of these fumes can cause immediate death.

The bottom line is that if you are sleeping on a mattress or pillow made from polyurethane foam, you are breathing in all of the chemicals the foam will release over its lifetime, and these could include chemicals such as toluene diisocyanate, methylene chloride, and formaldehyde. Many of these are considered potential carcinogens or have been associated with a number of adverse health effects.

Memory Polyurethane Foam

Many popular commercial mattresses advertise the use of visco-elastic (or "memory") foam as a selling point. This open-celled, temperature-sensitive, petroleum-based chemical polyurethane foam often claims origins in NASA research. Some of the ads I have seen make the veiled inference that it must be a good mattress if astronauts use it in space. This is of course absurd, since they are sleeping in weightless space, tethered so they don't float around the cabin. While it is formulated to alter its solid characteristics in response to body and room temperature, I believe NASA never actually used the product because of its chemical outgassing.

Technically, the aligned spherical cells of memory foam deform or soften in relationship to pressure and heat. When stress or weight are removed, the released cells return to their original configuration. Often referred to as visco-elastic foam, this describes the fact that at lower temperatures the foam is harder and more viscous, and is softer and more elastic at higher temperatures.

Visco-elastic foam differs from conventional polyurethane foam in that it uses a high-hydroxy polyol and different isocyanates. The formula for this material also utilizes specialty surfactants, cell-opening polyols, and additives, together with a unique manufacturing process, to create the "body-forming" characteristics so commonly described in mattress advertisements.

Latex Foam

The word "latex" can be confusing for consumers, because it has been used to describe both natural and synthetic products interchangeably, without adequate explanation. There are actually two types of latex: natural latex (also known as "natural rubber latex") and styrene-butadiene rubber (SBR, or "synthetic latex"). Latex mattress cores or paddings can also be created from a combination of natural and synthetic latex. These hybrid formulas are often referred to simply as "latex," leaving the consumer to guess the actual origins of the product. In Europe, manufacturers are required to provide information on mattress labels regarding the percentages of synthetic and natural latex used in a product. However, there is currently no law in the United States that requires such disclosure.

Natural rubber latex originates from the sap of rubber trees grown in areas around the equator, such as Sri Lanka, Malaysia, Africa and Indonesia. Brazil is also a major producer of natural rubber. The typical composition of raw natural latex is approximately 36 percent natural rubber, 0.3 percent amino acids, 1 percent neutral lipids, 1.6 percent proteins, 0.6 percent phospholipids, 1.5 percent carbohydrates, 0.5 percent salt, and 58.5 percent water. Natural rubber is a very stable raw material that benefits from the protective action of enzymes present in the juices of the rubber tree. These enzymes give the material its characteristic high flexibility in both hot and cold temperatures and its excellent long-term resilience.

Synthetic latex, or styrene-butadiene rubber, is created through the chemical polymerization of about 23 percent styrene and 77 percent butadiene. Chemicals, liquids, and gases are pumped continuously into reactors, which create, through catalyzation, the end product: artificial latex.

Both natural and synthetic latex use a number of chemical additives, such as natural soaps, zincs, sulfur, fatty acids, antioxidants, and accelerators that facilitate the heat curing (or "vulcanization") of the product. During the final phases of latex manufacturing, some manufacturers wash the finished cores numerous times to remove chemical additives that have not bonded during the foaming process.

Flame Retardants

Almost 35 years ago, due to deaths from fires caused by people smoking in bed, U.S. lawmakers passed regulations requiring that all mattresses be resistant to cigarette ignition. This means that today, mattress manufacturers are required to ensure that a cigarette will not set a mattress aflame. Mattress manufacturers met this flammability requirement by either treating the cover material with some type of chemical flame retardant or using a fire barrier made from noncombustible material. Polyurethane foam is extremely flammable, so it must be soaked in chemicals such as boric acid or polybrominated diphenyl ethers (PBDEs). Since this regulation was introduced in 1973, mattress fires have declined greatly, but many people question to what degree exposure to these chemical fire retardants have affected human health.

In 2004, a new mattress flammability law (AB603) was passed in California that significantly strengthened previous national flammability standards. This law requires manufacturers to ensure that mattresses sold in California are able to resist ignition from open flame, rather than just a smoldering cigarette. A similar version of this legislation has been adopted by the U.S. Consumer Product Safety Commission, and became effective throughout the United States on July 1, 2007.

While it is true that most mattress fires are more likely to start from open-flame sources such as candles, matches, or lighters, the legislation does not evaluate the long-term health risks associated with the chemical additives used to achieve the new flammability standard. And while I do not intend to minimize the suffering and death caused by mattress fires, such incidents involve hundreds, rather than millions, of consumers. Therefore, to protect hundreds, we are exposing the entire population of the United States to chemicals that have not been evaluated for their short- or long-term health risks. Many health experts and environmental activists believe that the potential health risks of the new law outweigh its benefits.

Organic mattresses generally meet flammability standards by using wool beneath the exterior cover fabric. Wool is a natural fire retardant and does not require any additional chemical treatments.

Just take a look at two of the chemicals most commonly used to reduce the flammability of conventional mattresses.

Boric Acid

The application of boric acid has become a standard method for reducing the flammability of cotton fibers. It is introduced to the fibers in the mixing machine, along with small amounts of oils and chemical surfactants. In order to ensure even distribution and adherence to the fibers, the boric acid is ground into a fine powder prior to application.

While boric acid is an ancient method of fireproofing cloth, it is also a known poisonous pesticide and insecticide. It is the primary ingredient in many bug sprays and flea-control products on the market today. When roaches, ants, fleas, and other bugs are exposed to this chemical, it kills them and their entire colony within three weeks.

Boric acid works as a desiccant. In other words, it kills bugs by removing moisture from their bodies, causing severe dehydration and affecting their electrolyte metabolism. Boric acid is also a stomach poison that can enter the body through ingestion, inhalation, or absorption through the skin.

The EPA warns of the potential for reproductive, developmental, and neurological damage in the use of boric acid. This chemical is associated with many known health risks, including genital damage, brain damage, anemia, infertility, birth defects, and death. At the very least, it can be extremely drying and irritating to the skin and lungs. Symptoms of boric acid poisoning include nausea, vomiting, diarrhea, headache, cold sweats, difficulty swallowing, difficulty breathing, muscle weakness, skin eruptions, skin discoloration, cardiac weakness, and coma.

The Agency for Toxic Substances and Disease Registry (a division of the Centers for Disease Control and Prevention) published a fact sheet to answer frequently asked questions about boron, which is the source of boric acid. In this report, the agency made the following comments about human exposure to boron:

"Breathing moderate levels of boron can result in irritation of the nose, throat, and eyes. Reproductive effects, such as low sperm count, were seen in men exposed to boron over the long term. Animal studies have shown effects on the lungs from breathing high levels of boron.

"Ingesting large amounts of boron over short periods of time can harm the stomach, intestines, liver, kidneys, and brain. Animal studies of ingestion of boron found effects on the testes in male animals. Birth defects were also seen in the offspring of female animals exposed during pregnancy.

"We don't know what the effects are in people from skin contact with boron. Animal studies have found skin irritation when boron was applied directly to the skin."

Polybrominated Diphenyl Ethers

Polybrominated diphenyl ethers, or PBDEs, belong to a class of chemicals introduced as a safer alternative to toxic polychlorinated biphenyls (PCBs) and polybrominated biphenyls (PBBs). However, recent scientific evidence suggests that amounts of PBDEs as small as one part per million can cause long-term behavioral alterations in experimental animals. Since PBDEs were commonly used in mattress manufacturing until January 2005, they are most likely part of the mattress you presently sleep on.

PBDEs may currently be found in a wide range of household products, from kids' pajamas to computers. Research shows they have been accumulating in the environment and in human bodies for the past several decades.

In 2003, a shocking report from the Environmental Working Group (EWG) analyzed the breast milk in women across the United States. The report concluded that "The average level of bromine-based fire retardants in the milk of 20 first-time mothers was 75 times the average found in recent European studies. Milk from two study participants contained the highest levels of fire retardants ever reported in the United States, and milk from several of the mothers in EWG's study had among the highest levels of these chemicals yet detected worldwide."

Recent studies have shown that these brominated compounds can interfere with the thyroid hormone, which is critical for the proper development of the brain and central nervous system in animals and humans. Baby mice exposed to PBDEs show permanent behavioral and memory problems, which worsen with age. Relatively recent reports also indicate that exposure to low concentrations of these chemicals may result in irreparable damage to the reproductive system.

The European Union banned two of the three most common PBDE formulations in 2004. In the U.S., California was the first state to take action against these dangerous chemicals, passing a law in 2004 to ban certain

PBDEs (however, due to lobbying by the chemical industry the law didn't take effect until 2008). Since California's ban, more states, including New York, Hawaii, and Oregon have taken action against PBDEs.

Water and Stain Repellents

Many mattress and mattress-pad retailers offer water- and stain-repellent treatments for their products to supposedly guard against damage to the mattress. Some retailers also offer to apply such treatments to untreated mattresses at an additional cost to the buyer.

One popular water- and stain-repellent treatment is DuPont's Teflon®, the same product used to prevent sticking on pots and pans. In the past few years, researchers have taken a closer look at the principal chemical component of Teflon: perfluorooctanoic acid (PFOA). According to the EPA, PFOA is a very persistent chemical. It has been found in both the environment and in the blood of people in the general population. PFOA has been linked to developmental delays and other adverse effects in laboratory animals. There is also concern about possible health effects to workers.

The Environmental Protection Agency's investigation into the persistence and effects of PFOA resulted in several large fines for DuPont. In December 2005, the EPA released a statement verifying that DuPont would be forced to pay a record $10.25 million fine for failing to tell the agency what the company knew about PFOA, including studies that found the substance in human blood, and said it should be considered "extremely toxic." According to the EPA's complaint, DuPont failed to submit a 1981 study that revealed PFOA was passed from pregnant employees to their fetuses. Company records showed that two of the five babies born to Teflon plant employees that year had eye and face defects similar to those found in newborn rats who were exposed to the chemical.

The EPA also stated that DuPont withheld the results from several 1997 studies regarding PFOA. One of these studies revealed that the rats died from inhaling chemicals related to PFOA. Another study found that high levels of PFOA were found in the blood of people living near the West Virginia plant where Teflon is made.

In addition to the federal fines, DuPont has also agreed to pay at least $107 million to settle the class-action lawsuit brought forth by the thousands of West Virginians and Ohioans who live near the Teflon plant.

Scotchgard™, a similar treatment made by 3M, uses a compound related to PFOA. Both 3M and DuPont went into negotiations with the EPA to fund studies that will evaluate the potential presence of PFOA and similar compounds in air, water, soils, sediments, and biota.

Adhesives

The fabrication of foam used in upholstered furniture and mattresses relies heavily on the use of adhesives. Historically, the adhesives used by foam manufacturers were based on 1,1,1-trichloroethane (TCA), an ozone-depleting substance. When production of TCA was banned in 1996, these industries converted mainly to adhesives based on methylene chloride, a suspected carcinogen. In April 2000, the Occupational Safety and Health Administration (OSHA) developed very stringent regulations on the use of methylene chloride. Therefore, many companies have been searching for alternative adhesive methods. Acetone-based adhesives and hot-melt production methods are two alternatives currently being incorporated into the production of foam for the mattress industry. Table 2 lists adhesives that

Table 2: Characteristics of Foam Mattress Adhesives

Adhesive	Classified as a VOC	Ozone Depleter	Hazards
TCA	No	Yes	Production banned due to environmental hazards
Methylene Chloride	No	No	Heavily regulated due to human health hazards such as dizziness, nausea, tingling in the extremities, skin reactions, and pulmonary dysfunction
Acetone Blends	Yes	No	Fire regulations
Hot Melt	No	No	Requires high temperature for application

are currently used in the fabrication of mattress foam and the potential hazards associated with each.

1,1,1-Trichloroethane-Based Adhesives

In the 1980s and early 1990s, most adhesives used by foam fabricators, upholstered-furniture manufacturers, and mattress manufacturers were based on TCA. However, in the 1990s, TCA was designated as a Class I ozone-depleting compound that destroys ozone in the upper atmosphere. Production of the chemical was banned in 1996 for that reason.

When TCA is released into the environment, it enters the air, where it lasts for about six years. Once in the air, this chemical may travel to the ozone layer, where it can be broken down by sunlight into chemicals that may reduce the ozone layer. It can also enter the environment through landfills and hazardous-waste sites, contaminating the surrounding soil and nearby surface water and groundwater.

Methylene Chloride-Based Adhesives

In 1996, after the ban on TCA production, foam manufacturers turned to the chemical methylene chloride in their production processes. Methylene chloride is a colorless liquid with a mild, sweet odor. It is also referred to as dichloromethane. This synthetic chemical is not known to damage the ozone layer as TCA does; however, it may have significant negative effects on human health.

According to the Agency for Toxic Substance and Disease Registry, breathing in large amounts of methylene chloride can cause unsteadiness, dizziness, and nausea. Exposure can also cause tingling or numbness in the fingers and toes. Even exposure to smaller amounts of methylene chloride may cause a person to become less attentive and less accurate in tasks requiring hand-eye coordination. Skin contact with methylene chloride causes burning and redness.

Health experts have not yet determined if methylene chloride causes cancer in humans. But in animal studies, mice that were exposed to large amounts of methylene chloride for extended periods presented an increased risk of cancer. The World Health Organization, the Department of Health and Human Services, and the EPA have all issued statements that methylene chloride is a probable cancer-causing agent in humans. Because of this, the Occupational Safety and Health Administration (OSHA) has set strict limits on the amount of methylene chloride employees can be exposed to in the workplace. Therefore, many companies are again looking for alternative adhesives to use in mattresses and other bedding.

Acetone-Based Adhesives

Acetone-based chemicals are currently being considered by companies searching for alternatives to TCA and methylene chloride. However, acetone-based adhesives are not without environmental and health hazards of their own. These chemicals have a very low flash point, meaning that companies that use these chemicals must take measures to minimize the chance of fire or explosion. Some formulations based on acetone also contain other chemicals, such as hexane, heptane, and mineral spirits, that can be hazardous to human health. Although significant studies have not been performed, acetone-based adhesives may be classified as VOCs, and some may be relatively toxic.

Hot-Melt Adhesives

An additional adhesive alternative is the hot-melt adhesive, which is applied to foam products with a special spray gun that heats the resins in the adhesive to 300°F or higher so they can flow freely. The applied adhesive then quickly cools and sets. In the mattress-manufacturing sector, hot-melt adhesives pose the least risk to both human and environmental health. However, their use requires a significant investment in materials and equipment from companies that are currently using chemicals such as methylene chloride.

Formaldehyde

Formaldehyde is commonly found in both indoor and outdoor air. It occurs naturally as a by-product of combustion and decaying animal or plant wastes, and is synthetically or commercially produced for a wide range of industrial uses and products.

Formaldehyde finds its way into mattresses because it is routinely used in the manufacture of textiles, wood products, and some adhesives. It is used frequently in the form of a plastic resin to enhance the appearance and wrinkling properties of fabrics that can be used as mattress tickings, or it can be added to the yarns when they are spun.

When individuals are exposed to formaldehyde levels over 0.1 part per million (ppm), they may experience watery or burning eyes; irritation of the nose, throat, or skin; coughing; wheezing; and nausea. Formaldehyde was classified as a known human carcinogen in 2004 by the International Agency for Research on Cancer (IARC), and the U.S. Environmental Protection Agency (EPA) considers it a probable human carcinogen under conditions of unusually high or prolonged exposure.

The GREENGUARD Environmental Institute offers a certification for commercial products that have been submitted for toxic emission testing and met their various emission criteria. For example, for a mattress to be GREENGUARD certified, its formaldehyde emissions cannot exceed 0.02 ppm.

The only mattresses that have ever been certified by this organization are those made by OMI and sold by the national organic catalog company Lifekind® Products, Inc. and other environmentally conscious retailers.

Solvents

Solvents show up in mattress emissions because they are critical ingredients in many of the adhesives used to bond together mattress layers and wood frames. Solvents are also present in the lubricants and cleaning agents used on factory equipment, and can often be found in packaging materials.

Table 3: Health Hazards of Common Mattress Solvents

Chemical	Health Hazards
Styrene	Toxic to the lungs, liver, and brain
Isopropylbenzene	Respiratory tract irritant
Limonene	Respiratory tract irritant
Trimethylbenzene	Carcinogen and neurotoxin
Nitrobenzene	Known to cause testicular degeneration and methemoglobinemia
Ethylbenzene	Toxic to the liver, kidneys, and brain
Dichlorobenzene	Carcinogen

One of the most common solvents used today in the mattress industry is based on methylene chloride (METH), which is a suspected carcinogen. Alternatives are available, and some manufacturers have changed to safer forms of bonding that use non-METH hot-melt adhesives.

In 2000, an independent scientific organization known as Anderson Laboratories ran tests to identify the chemicals present in standard conventional mattresses. The chemicals they identified were primarily solvents such as styrene, isopropylbenzene, limone, trimethylbenzene, nitrobenzene, ethylbenzene, and dichlorobenzene. Each of these chemicals is associated with a host of human health conditions. Table 3 lists each of the chemicals and their associated health hazards.

Chapter Three

Is Your Mattress Safe?
(How Long Can You Hold
Your Breath?)

"Sleep is the golden chain that ties health and our bodies together."
—Thomas Dekker

THE FOLLOWING REMARKS are from consumers who experienced adverse health effects after purchasing new mattresses. These comments are from people all over North America whose symptoms are very disturbing—and very similar. They represent a fraction of the people whom I have spoken to regarding the health reactions they have associated with their mattresses and bedding. A far more extensive list of consumer comments can be found at the consumer bulletin board www.chem-tox.com.

"I'm actually going on my third mattress with this retailer. The retailer tells me that no one else has experienced any problems with the mattress. All I know is that I have not been feeling myself since I purchased the mattress. I've experienced headaches, dizziness, memory loss, and tiredness!"—A.M.K., Branford, CT

"After purchasing our new mattress, I awoke the first night at midnight feeling anxious and with a stomach ache. My symptoms progressed to muscle-shaking (hands, legs, even my back), headache, and dizziness."—A.S., Pacific Palisades, CA

"The minute the mattress was unwrapped, I noticed a strong chemical smell and I immediately felt stuffed up, like I was getting a cold. I couldn't sleep on it, and the smell permeated the house making my family feel sick. The department store was very apologetic and said they have never had a complaint like this before."—D.H., Victoria, Canada

"About 30 days ago, we purchased a memory-foam mattress. Suddenly, our skin has become very itchy; our throats are sore; we have broken out in red rashes where we have contact with the mattress and pillows; difficulty breathing, etc. I never thought that we could get sick from our bed."—R.T., Providence, RI

"After receiving my new mattress I began to feel foggy, irritable, itchy, and I felt a tightness in my lungs. The symptoms increased until I removed the mattress from our house and took a shower."—S.M., Portland, OR

"I purchased a new factory-made mattress. It had a horrible strong odor like mildew and mothballs. I developed respiratory problems and chest pains."—C.T., Seattle, WA

Janine Phariss of Phoenix, Arizona, and her husband know firsthand the health problems associated with modern commercial mattresses. In their recent search for a new mattress, Janine and her husband found that each one they tried "stank to high heaven." After purchasing a popular brand and bringing it home, they experienced health effects ranging from annoying to severe. "My husband has had several headaches, and severe pain in his neck and shoulder," said Janine. "My husband is one of those folks with a very healthy constitution, so for him to get a rash was strange to say the least."

Janine was also plagued by health problems. "I've had headaches, and I don't normally get them. I've had rashes on my legs, swollen tonsils, and body aches." Janine and her husband also complained of feeling "foggy" in the morning when they would wake up. "He got better when he was at work after a while, and I seemed to feel a little better by about 4 p.m., or anytime I was out of the house or had the door closed to the bedroom," she said.

Debora Rouse of South Milwaukee, Wisconsin, has faced one ailment after another in reaction to the chemicals in her pillows and mattress topper. In early 2005, Debora and her husband purchased a pillow top that was advertised to "add luxury to your ordinary mattress" and "provide an extravagant sleeping surface that customizes to comfort your entire body."

Debora recently described their experience. "My husband's face swelled up, with his lower lip getting huge. I developed hives, with horrible itching and a sinus infection that just won't go away. As an experiment, I tried sleeping in our guest room for a few nights and my hives started to resolve, but not my sinus infection, even after being on antibiotics for a week. I also had a reaction of facial swelling of my eyes and lower lip, weeks after purchasing the topper and pillows. I hadn't actually slept on the pillow, I only used it for support when sitting up reading. Thinking back, my face swelling occurred on the one night I actually slept on the pillow. My eyes would burn when I would sit up and read in bed, as I often do, using the memory-foam pillows for support. I also experienced intense fatigue. My energy level has dropped to the point where EVERYTHING is a major effort."

These reactions are similar to those experienced by many people who are exposed to chemically laden mattresses. Linda B., of British Columbia, Canada, experienced headaches and sinus problems, and felt that her throat was closing every time she slept on her new mattress. "What is so strange is usually I don't have headaches or any allergies. But for sure my headaches, sinus problem, and closing of the throat are from the new beds, because during the 'in-between new bed times' my head clears. I'm also fine once I've been outside for an hour or so."

Some people are simply more sensitive to the chemicals and gases that are used in the making of modern mattresses. This sensitivity can cause some of the immediate symptoms, such as rashes, headaches, breathing difficulties, and blurred vision, that have been described by people who have recently purchased a new mattress. Others may experience side effects such as fatigue, nausea, or difficulty concentrating, which are more difficult to link to chemical exposure.

Prior to the studies done for this book, there has been very little published on short-term VOC emissions from modern mattresses. While some short-term emission studies and industry-sponsored studies have been performed on mattresses and polyurethane foam, most have been conducted by commercial firms promoting the use of specific raw materials or formulas. There have been no coordinated research efforts. One of the most significant limitations of these studies is that they are short term, conducted at temperatures other than body temperature. It is impossible to simulate the actual health effects on any given individual over time unless a study could be performed to measure emission levels under conditions that are more typical of one's long-term sleeping environment.

Mattress Emission Studies

Here is a summary of some of the most recent studies that have been performed on VOC emissions and mattress components:

- Several commercial studies performed by Nitroil Performance Chemical, in Hamburg, Germany, have analyzed VOC emission levels in molded foams and lower-density slabstock polyurethane foams. The researchers found that these components emit harmful VOCs such as triethylenediamine and dimethylaminoethyl, as well as flame retardants such as tris(2-chloroisopropyl)phosphate, tris(dichloroethylisopropyl)phosphate, and tris(chloroethylisopropyl)phosphate.

- A short-term study sponsored by the Sleep Products Safety Council tested six mattresses and their individual components in an attempt to characterize and identify emissions. The VOCs mentioned in their study were acetaldehyde and n-hexanal, probably coming from the glue used on corner sections, and formaldehyde, most likely emitting from the textile materials. They also noted "low levels of 2,4- and 2,6 toluene diisocyanate, which are typical emissions from polyurethane foam components." (The Sleep Products Safety Council is an arm of the International Sleep Products Association, which is composed of over 700 wholesalers, retailers, and manufacturers of mattresses and foundations, representing approximately 80 percent of the industry.)

- In 1999, Anderson Laboratories, Inc., in West Hartford, Vermont, conducted emission tests on five crib mattresses to determine the potential for respiratory toxicity of mattress emissions. Using gas chromatography and mass spectrometry to identify respiratory inhalants, researchers documented chemical emissions such as styrene, isopropylbenzene, limonene, trimethylbenzene, nitrobenzene, ethylbenzene, 1,3-p menthadiene, b-ocimene, and dichlorobenzene. However, due to limitations of the analysis equipment used, researchers were unable to identify many of the chemicals emitted with at least 85 percent certainty.

The Anderson crib study helped to underscore the importance of the sleeping environment for children. Because children breathe faster than adults, they are particularly vulnerable to the chemical exposure.

A study published in the *Archives of Environmental Health* examined the health effects of sleeping on a conventional mattress. Researchers exposed groups of male Swiss-Webster mice to the emissions of several brands of mattresses for two one-hour periods. They then tested the animals for respiratory frequency, pattern, and airflow velocity. Their research revealed that the emissions of four of the mattresses caused various combinations of upper-airway irritation, such as sensory irritation, pulmonary irritation, and decreases in mid-expiratory airflow velocity.

A traditional mattress with wire springs and fiber padding caused sensory irritation in more than half of all breaths taken. This mattress also caused pulmonary irritation in 23 percent of breaths, and a decrease in airflow in 11 percent of breaths. The largest decrease in airflow occurred with the mattress that was topped with a polyurethane foam pad and vinyl cover. All of the mattresses in the study caused pulmonary irritation. Using gas chromatography and mass spectrometry, the researchers identified potential respiratory irritants, such as styrene, isopropylbenzene, and limonene, in the emissions of one of the polyurethane foam mattresses. Some of the mattresses emitted mixtures of volatile chemicals that had the potential to cause respiratory tract irritation and decrease airflow velocity in mice.

Now consider this: The study's authors also performed a similar experiment using organic cotton padding. This research produced very different results. When the mice in the study were exposed to this bedding, they presented *increases* in both respiratory rate and volume of air inhaled and exhaled with each breath. The researchers found that organic cotton bedding actually *improved* the respiratory health of the study subjects.

People who experience short-term, acute reactions to their chemically based mattresses may have an easier time linking their symptoms to their mattresses, but what about the long-term side effects of prolonged exposure to chemicals and toxins? While the volume of new-mattress outgassing does lessen over time (the worst of it being emitted in the first 60 days), I believe it never really stops. All chemical components decay over time and emit various substances during the process. Witness the film formed on the inside of a car's windshield. It exists for many years after you buy your car. This film is composed primarily of chemicals outgassing from the polyurethane products used to make the car's interior. The windshield provides a convenient and observable collection surface.

This brings us to the discussion of a concept called "BQL," or "Below Quantifiable Levels." This is the point in analytical analysis when the substance being tested is below the amount that the testing equipment can discern. BQL does not mean no chemicals are present, just that the testing procedure or equipment is not sensitive enough to register their presence. The risks we expose ourselves to from long-term exposure to very low chemical levels is currently unknown. Hopefully studies now underway will shed more light on the subject.

Nicole Armand, of Eugene, Oregon, was also shocked to discover the health risks associated with modern chemically based mattresses. A few years ago, Nicole and her husband purchased a new innerspring mattress from one of the major brands. The first night they slept on it, Nicole experienced a mild seizure, but was unaware of its cause. For the next two years, Nicole had seizures that were increasingly severe. Her doctors finally found a medication that helped to control them, but neither they nor Nicole uncovered the link between her seizures and her mattress. Over the years, she also developed fibromyalgia and chronic fatigue syndrome. Unfortunately, she has only just recently begun to suspect that her health problems were likely brought on by exposure to her new mattress. "We didn't let it offgas, as we did not know any better, but I do remember the odor of the mattress when it was new, and to this day I still suffer so badly that I cannot work anymore. Could a mattress be the culprit to my downward-spiraling health conditions?" she asked.

Nicole still has the same mattress, but no longer sleeps on it. "I am sure it is done offgassing, but the damage has already been done," she added.

Eric Sutton, of Ashburn, Virginia, is another consumer who is all too familiar with the potential health effects associated with synthetically produced mattresses. "For our anniversary, my wife and I decided to trade our old mattress in for a popular memory-foam sleep system that we saw in a local national mall store," he said in a recent interview. "We purchased the top-of-the-line king-size mattress with additional pillow top, as well as the recommended foundation (to replace the normal box spring). We also splurged and got two of the memory-foam pillows as well. In all, we spent over $4,000."

Eric and his wife thought they were purchasing a mattress that would *improve* their sleep and overall health. Instead, they found the opposite to be true.

"The mattress couldn't be delivered until the following week, but we were able to take the pillows home immediately. It was late when we got home from the store, so as we got ready for bed, we unboxed the pillows and immediately noticed the horrible smell of the material," said Eric. He explained that he and his wife were almost to the point of gagging from the odor of their new "top-of-the-line" pillows. "There was a sticker on the pillow that stated that the pillow would have an odor, but that it was harmless and that after a few days it would dissipate. I remember not being comfortable with the pillow on the first night, and woke the next morning with a severe headache and a stiff neck. I didn't think much of it at the time, and continued to sleep with the pillow for a few more days before ditching it and returning to my 'normal' pillow."

A week later, when Eric's new mattress arrived, he found it to be extremely comfortable. "It supported every inch of my body without pressure points," he said. However, just like the pillow, Eric's new mattress emitted a horrible odor: "It filled the entire house with a chemical smell that was impossible to ignore." The very next day, Eric woke up experiencing tremendous pain in every joint in his body, including his neck, shoulders, elbows, back, hips, and knees. He also experienced severe muscle pain around those joints, and significant weakness.

As the owner of a personal fitness studio who works out every day, Eric's first assumption was that he had over-trained the day before. But as the days went on, his pain got worse. "It got so bad that I couldn't move without excruciating pain, and it was so debilitating, I couldn't go to work because I couldn't roll myself over in bed, let alone walk up and down stairs or lift any weight heavier than five pounds."

After a few days of staying in bed and "feeling like I wanted to die," Eric finally went to the doctor with unbearable pain and muscle fatigue throughout his entire body. His doctor ran all sorts of blood tests for conditions such as Lyme disease, mononucleosis and strep throat, but they came back negative. Eric spent the next week in bed on painkillers, unable to move.

After six weeks with the new mattress, Eric was still feeling horrible, but he had not made the connection between his symptoms and his mattress … until the night he stayed away from home. He woke up the next morning and immediately noticed that his pain and stiffness weren't quite as bad. "Immediately things began to click," he said. "I returned to my home the following day, and after just one night's sleep on the memory-foam mattress, I returned to feeling completely miserable." Eric knew the return of his symptoms was somehow linked to his new mattress. After doing some research on the Internet, he stumbled upon a website that was filled with reports from others who were experiencing similar health effects. "Needless to say, I started sleeping in our guest room until we returned the mattress and pillows."

Immediately after Eric and his wife returned their mattress and pillows, he started feeling better. It took about three weeks for most of his physical symptoms to dissipate. About eight weeks after returning the mattress, Eric was back to his normal self and working out with full effort.

Potential Health Hazards of Memory-Foam Mattresses

Eric's story is not an isolated one, and you're about to understand why. Recently, I had one of the popular memory-foam mattresses tested by a reputable laboratory using methods that complied with ASTM Standards D-5116-97 and D-56670-01 92,8 and the EPA's ETV protocol (9). The entire mattress was placed in a sealed stainless-steel environmental chamber, where chemical emissions were collected, measured and analyzed over a 96-hour period. The VOC measurements were taken by gas chromatography together with mass spectrometric detection (GC/MS). While some of the chemicals detected cannot be identified with 100 percent certainty, mass spectral libraries made available from NISST, the USEPA, and the National Institutes of Health (NIH) were used to characterize compounds. Combined with the testing laboratories' own databases, these data provide a high level of identification reliability.

In total, the memory-foam mattress emitted 61 VOC chemicals. Here is the list:

1,2,4-Methenoazulene, decahydro-1,5,5,8a tetra methyl

1,2-Propanediol (Propylene Glycol)

1,4-Dioxane

1,6-Octadiene, 7 -methyl-3-methylene (Myrcene)

1-Butanol (N-Butyl alcohol)

1-Dodecene

1-Hexanol,2-ethyl

1-Propanol, 2-chloro-*

2-Butanol, 3-methyl

2-Pentenal, 2-methyl

2-Propanol (Isopropanol)

2-Propanol, 1,3-diehloro-

2-Propanol, 1-(2-Dropenyloxy)

2-Propanol, 1-[1-methyl-2-(2-propenyloxy) ethoxy*

Azulene, 1,2,3,4,5,6, 7,8-oetahydro-1,4-dimethyl-7- 12.6 (1-methylethylidene)

Benzaldehyde

Benzene, 1,2,4-trimethyl

Benzene, 1,3-diehloro

Benzene, 1,4-diehloro

Benzene, 1-methylethyl (Cumene)

Bicyclo[3.1.1]hept-2-ene-2-carbox-aldehyde

Bicyclo[3.1.1]heptan-3-one, 2,6,6-trimethyl-.1a,2b,5a*

Chlorobenzene

Cyclohexane, 1, 1-dimethyl-2-propyl*

Cyclohexane, octyl*

Cyclohexasiloxane, dodecamethyl*

Cyclohexene, 1-methyl-4-(1-methylethylidene)*

Cyclopentasiloxane, decamethyl

Cyclotetrasiloxane, octamethyl

Cyclotrisiloxane, hexamethyl

Decane, 3-methyl

Decane, 5-methyl*

Dodecane

Dodecane, 3-methyl

Heptylcyclohexane*

Hexanal

Hexasiloxane, tetradecamethyl (8CI9CI)*

Limonene (Dipentene; 1-Methyl-4-1 methylethyl cyclohexene)

Longifolene

Naphthalene

Naphthalene, decahydro-*

Naphthalene, decahydro-2-methyl*

Pentasiloxane, dodecamethyl*

Phenol, 4-(1-methylpropYI)-*

Pinene, a (2,6,6- Trimethyl-bieyelor3.1.1]hept-2-ene)

Pinene, p (6,6-Dimethyl-2-meth-ylene bieyelo[3.1.1]heptane)

Propane, 1,2,3-trichloro

Propane, 1,2-dichloro

Propanoic acid, 2,2-dimethyl-, 2-ethylhexyl ester*

Silane, trichloro(chloromethyl)-*

Silanediol, dimethyl-*

Styrene

TXIB (2,2,4-Trimethyl-1,3-pentanediol diisobutyrate)

Tetrasiloxane, decamethyl

Toluene (Methylbenzene)

Trisiloxane, octamethyl*

Undecane

Undecane, 2,6-dimethyl

Undecane, 2-methyl

Xylene (para and/or meta)

c- Decahydronaphthalene

*Indicates NIST/EPAINIH best library match only based on retention time and mass spectral characteristics with a probability of > 80 percent. '1 'i1. ~ 5. Individual volatile organic compounds are calibrated relative to toluene. All individual VOCs detected met the criteria of less than 1/100 the ACGIH-established threshold limit value (TL V) and/or less than percent the CA chronic reference exposure level (CREL). Quantifiable level is 0.04 I1g based on a standard 18 L air collection volume.

It is not within the scope of this book to advise the reader as to any potential health risks from short-, long-term or chronic low-level exposure to these specific chemicals. However, I believe it is extremely important that some kind of label or warning information should inform consumers that outgassing from memory-foam products can expose them to chemicals such as those listed on the previous page. Several of the chemicals on this list have been widely recognized as harmful by the California Health and Welfare Agency, the International Agency on Research of Cancer (IARC), and the EPA, yet consumers take these mattresses into their bedrooms unaware that their health may be jeopardized because they have never been made aware of the potential risks.

Human health risks for the chemicals mentioned in this chapter and throughout this book can be found on many websites. One of my favorites is IRIS (the Integrated Risk Information System), operated by the EPA's Office of Research and Development and the National Center for Environmental Assessment. This database is intended to provide consumers with a source of nontechnical, reliable information on chemicals, and can be found on the web at www.epa.gov/iris/index.html. Also, Scorecard is a great source for finding out about toxins in your local community, as well as individual chemical profiles, which can be found at www.scorecard.org. I also use the Agency for Toxic Substances and Disease Registry (ATSDR), which can be found at www.atsdr.cdc.gov.

Please note that even though you may find Internet sites that claim to sell chemical-free mattresses and bedding, there is no such thing. In fact, I do not believe there are any consumer products that are completely free of chemicals. If a company is making that claim, you should ask for a letter or copy of the testing documentation to verify its representation. And even though organic mattresses greatly reduce your chemical exposures, some level of chemical exposure is unavoidable. In truth, there is no place I could recommend that you could sleep where you would not be exposed to some level of chemical exposure (see discussion of the **Avoidance or Substitution Rule** on page 77).

There are mattresses and bedding products that you can purchase that will lower your exposure to chemicals significantly. For instance, the mattresses manufactured by Organic Mattresses, Inc. (OMI) and sold by the catalog company Lifekind®, Inc. (www.lifekind.com) and other organically conscious retailers throughout the United States are not only made in the only third-party certified organic production facility, but they have also been independently tested for VOC exposures, and their mattresses have met all of the low-level emission requirements of the GREENGUARD Environmental Institute.

Volatile Organic Compounds

Volatile organic compounds (VOCs) are emitted as gases from certain solids or liquids. They can be found in everything from underarm deodorants, to paints and sealants, and household cleaning products. VOCs include a variety of chemicals, such as benzene, toluene, methylene, chloride, formaldehyde, xylene, ethylene glycol, texanol, and 1,3-butadiene. Many of these chemicals have been associated with short- and long-term adverse health effects. They are a major concern of the EPA and state air quality boards all over the United States.

VOCs are gases that vaporize easily at room temperature. They are known as "organic" because their chemical structures contain at least one carbon atom. VOCs are emitted by a wide array of products. Emission sources include perfumes, printing inks, mothballs, gasoline, cleaning supplies, pesticides, newspaper, carpets and other building materials, pressed-wood furniture, air fresheners, solvents, glues and adhesives, sealants, cosmetics, office equipment such as copiers and printers, correction fluids and carbonless copy paper, tobacco smoke, permanent markers, and photographic solutions. All of these products can release VOCs while you are using them, and, to some degree, when they are stored.

In the case of mattresses, VOCs are emitted from the fibers, foams, adhesives, fire retardants, and other additives that are used in mattress construction. Sleepers are exposed to these gases intimately and continuously throughout the night. This exposure subjects sleepers to a variety of unanticipated health risks and reactions, especially in those who are particularly sensitive to chemical emissions.

Most VOCs have no discernable odor, color, or smell. In fact, they are usually detected only by sophisticated laboratory-analysis techniques that utilize processes such as gas chromatography, flame ionization, mass spectrometry, and infrared spectroscopy. However, even with these sophisticated techniques, some VOC releases are too low for characterization.

A number of VOCs do produce a distinguishable odor; however, depending upon their molecular structure, they may have a citrus or fruity odor, or they may smell like oil, gasoline, almonds, or mothballs. The amine catalysts used in the production of polyurethane foam smell distinctly like fish. Carbon disulphide, on the other hand, smells like rotten eggs. These gases are emitted in the manufacturing of synthetic latex.

VOCs are responsible for the distinctive "new mattress" smell, similar to the "new car smell" in the automobile industry. In a study conducted by Scientific Instrument Services, of Ringoes, New Jersey, over 50 VOCs were identified in an air sample obtained from a new car. The air sample, collected first thing in the morning, was found to contain the toxic compound toluene, as well as numerous other VOCs that may have outgassed from the automobile's interior or from its associated exhaust fumes. Other VOCs were also detected that were related to cleaning and lubricating compounds used on the automobile. As the temperature increased in the car throughout the day, concentrations of these compounds also increased, together with the formation of new chemical gases such as styrene, benzene, and the antioxidant compound BHT. These benzene derivatives are common in gasoline, paints, and carpeting, whereas BHT is common in treatments for leather and vinyl. This study also found that although the VOCs present in new automobiles decreased over time, they probably never completely disappear, and worsen when exposed to higher temperatures.

The EPA's Total Exposure Assessment Methodology (TEAM) studies found levels of about a dozen common VOCs to be two to five times higher inside homes than outside, regardless of whether the homes were located in rural or industrial areas. Additional TEAM studies indicate that while people are using products containing VOCs, they can expose themselves and others to high pollutant levels much like secondhand smoke, and that elevated concentrations can persist in the air long after product use is discontinued.

At present, not much is known about the extent of symptoms or health effects that can occur from exposure to VOCs in the home. Unfortunately, studies looking into the effects of VOC emissions are limited. Therefore, it is difficult to make direct comparisons between studies, because one study may find one set of emissions while another study finds a different set.

Avoidance or Substitution Rule

Throughout my life, my philosophy has always been to simply avoid as many chemicals as possible.

If you cannot avoid a product that is high in chemical exposures, at least select a safer substitute or an alternative product.

For instance, if you desire the comfort of a memory-foam-type mattress such as the one described above, check out similar products made from natural rubber and organic materials. Here is a summary of the test results of these two types of products:

The emissions from the memory-foam mattress tested contained a total of 61 different chemical compounds. The total chemical emissions from these VOCs within the first four hours of testing was 7,958.10 micrograms (ug)/units per hour.

For comparison, I tested one of our natural rubber organic mattresses using these same methods. The total VOC emissions for this mattress during the same time period was 412 ug/units per hour. The OMI natural rubber mattress produced 95 percent less chemical emissions, and the chemicals themselves were generally safer. After 48 hours, the total emissions for the OMI natural rubber organic mattress was down to 127 ug/units per hour—96 percent lower than the 3,632.10 ug/units per hour coming from the memory-foam mattress.

The nature of the chemical compounds is also different for the two mattresses tested. After 24 hours, the OMI natural rubber organic mattress showed very small amounts of six chemicals: hexanol, 2-ethyl; benzothiazole; limonene; longifolene; nonyl aldehyde; and pinene. These chemicals most likely originated from the bio-soaps used to clean the wool, or possibly from the absorption of naturally occurring airborne substances in proximity to where the cotton was grown. These very low levels typically outgas in a fairly short period of time (four to eight hours, or days, not months or years), and based on the independent laboratory findings, represent a much more healthful option for people seeking the comfort of a latex mattress.

To further describe these six chemicals: hexanol, 2-ethyl occurs naturally in food, and is a component of several essential oils and aromas, such as apple, strawberry, and lavender. Benzothiazole also occurs naturally in fruits and vegetables, and while it is used to facilitate the natural-rubber vulcanizing process, derivatives of benzothiazole have also been shown to have anti-cancer and anti-dementia properties, in addition to being used to treat multiple sclerosis and other diseases. Limonene is a biodegradable solvent occurring in nature as the main component of citrus-peel oil. Longifolene is a naturally occurring oil extracted from pine-tree resin, and is often found in scented and aromatherapy products. Nonyl aldehyde, like limonene, is a major component of lemon-peel oil. Pinene occurs naturally in a variety of plants, fruits, and vegetables, such as carrots, tomatoes, and celery. It is also used as a fragrance in many consumer products. All six of these chemicals have been approved by the FDA for use as food additives and flavoring agents.

At higher levels of exposure, several of these chemicals can produce unhealthy reactions. However, I am confident that the low levels present and their rapid dissolution do not pose a problem. While it would be ideal to have zero levels of these (or any) chemicals present, if wool wasn't washed or packaging materials weren't used, it could introduce another whole group of potential contaminants. As I mentioned earlier, nothing in the world is truly chemical free.

Again, for comparison, **after 24 hours**, emissions from the memory-foam mattress tested 44 chemicals still present:

1,2-Propanediol (Propylene Glycol)

1, 6-Octadiene, 7 -methyl-3-meth-ylene (Myrcene)

1-Butanol (N-Butyl alcohol)1-Dodecene

1-Hexanol

2-ethyl, 2-Butanol, 3-methyl 2-Pentenal, 2-methyl, 2-Propanol (Isopropanol)

2-Propanol, 1,3-diehloro-, 2-Propanol, 1-(2-Dropenyloxy)

2-Propanol, 1-[1-methyl-2-(2-propenyloxy) ethoxy]

Benzene, 1,4-diehloro

Benzene, 1-methylethyl (Cumene, Bicyclo[3.1.1]hept-2-ene':2-carboxaldehyde Bicyclo[3.1.1]heptan-3-one, 2,6,6-trimethyl-.1a,2b,5a, Cyclohexane

1, 1-dimethyl-2-propyl

Cyclohexane, octyl,
   Cyclohexasiloxane,
   dodecamethyl
Cyclotetrasiloxane, octamethyl
Cyclotrisiloxane hexamethyl
Decane, 3-methyl, Dodecane, 3-
   methyl
Hexasiloxane, tetradecamethyl
   (8CI9CI), Limonene (Dipentene;
   1-Methyl-4-1 methylethyl cyclo-
   hexene)
Longifolene
Naphthalene
Naphthalene, decahydro-
Naphthalene, decahydro-2-methyl
Pentasiloxane, dodecamethyl

Pinene, a
Pinene, b
Propane, 1,2,3-triehloro
Propane, 1,2-dichloro
Propanoic acid, 2,2-dimethyl-,
   2-ethylhexyl ester
Silane, trichloro(chloromethyl)-
Silanediol, dimethyl-
Styrene
Tetrasiloxane, decamethyl
Undecane, Undecane, 2,6-dimethyl
Undecane, 2-methyl, c-
   Decahydronaphthalene
1,2,4-Methanoazulene
   decahydro-1,5,5,8a tetra methyl

Several of these chemicals, such as benzene, propane, styrene, and naphthalene, are recognized as possible Class C human carcinogens by the EPA, as well as other organizations. Naphthalene, the main ingredient in mothballs, has been associated with hemolytic anemia in infants, as well as liver and neurological damage in adults who have been exposed through inhalation or dermal contact. In addition, exposure to many of the chemicals listed above has been associated with irritation of the skin, eyes, mucous membranes, and gastrointestinal system. Additionally, exposures have been reported to produce headache, fatigue, depression, hearing loss, and peripheral neuropathy.

The website www.chem-tox.com provides a bulletin board where consumers can post health reactions they have had from chemical-based mattresses. The site is replete with anecdotal evidence, as well as extensive technical information in the form of chemical database reviews.

Chemical Exposures from a Typical Innerspring/Pillow-Top Mattress

Using the same reputable laboratory and chamber testing methods used for the memory-foam mattress (ASTM Standards D 5116-97 and D-56670-01 92,8 and EPA's ETV protocol [9]), a typical innerspring/pillow-top mattress emitted 39 VOC chemicals.

Here is a list of those chemicals:

1,2-Propanediol (Propylene glycol),

1-Pentanol,4-methyl-2-propyl (9C1)*

2,6-Di-tert-butyl-4-methyphenol (BHT)

2-Dodecene, (Z)-8C19C1*

3-Ethyl-3-methylheptane

3-isopropoxy-1,1,17,7,7-hexam-ethyl-3,5,5-tris (trimethyl-siloxy)tetrasiloxane*

5-Ethyldecane*

Cyclohexasiloxane dodecamethyl*

Cyclohexasiloxane decamethyl

Decane, 2,3,5,8-tetramethyl*

Decane 2,4-dimethyl*

Decane 3,6-dimethyl (8C19C1)

Decane, 4-methyl*

Decane, 5-methyl*

Dodecane, Dodecane 4-methyl*

Dodecane 5-methyl*

Ethene, 1,1,2,2-tetrachloro (tetra-chloroethylene)

Heptane, 2,2,4,6,6-pentamethyl (8C19C1)

Heptane 2,2,6,6-tetramethyl

Heptane,4-propyl

Heptane 5-ethyl-2,2,3-tribethyl*

Nonane, 2,3-dimethyl*

Nonane, 3,7-dimethyl*

Octane, 2,2-dimethyl*

Octane, 3,4 6-trimethyl*

Octane, 2,5,6-triimethyl* (9C1)

Octane, 3,3-dimethyl

Pinene a (2,6,6-Trimethyl-bicyclo [3.1.1.] hept-2-ene)

Propylene Carbonate*

Tetradecane

Tridecane

Tridecane, 5-propyl*

Undecane

Undecane 3-methyl*

Undecane 5,7-dimethyl (8C1)*

Undecane 5-methylene*

indicates NIST/NIH best library match only based on retention time and mass spectral characteristics with a probability of greater than 80 percent individual volatile organic compounds are calibrated relative to toluene. Quantifiable level is 0.04 upbased on a standard 18 L air collection volume.

As stated earlier in this chapter, it is not my intent to delve too deeply into the potential hazards of the specific chemicals mentioned above, but a few are of obvious concern. Tetrachloroethylene is listed within California's Proposition 65 as a carcinogen; the ATSDR and the EPA are also concerned that it may be a developmental toxicant. The EPA considers this chemical of possible concern as a gastrointestinal, liver, and kidney toxicant, and the ATSDR mentions it as a potential neurotoxicant.

Propylene glycol, a common ingredient in personal-care products, has been declared an illegal ingredient in the European Union because it is suspected of reproductive and developmental toxicity, as well as being a respiratory toxicant capable of producing irritation to the nasal passages, throat, and lungs.

For an outgassing comparison, an OMI innerspring mattress padded with certified organic cotton and organic wool was tested by the same laboratory using the same method. (The construction of the two mattresses are not identical, but they both use innersprings and paddings.)

If you prefer an innerspring-style mattress and apply my *Avoidance or Substitution Rule* in your evaluation, compare the following information:

The outgassing from the OMI innerspring mattress emitted the following chemicals: decanal and nonyl aldehyde (nonanal). These chemicals probably originated from the soaps used to clean the wool, and/or from normal airborne substances that can be absorbed by cotton and wool during their growth cycles. The decanal in this case probably came from the outgassing of citrus oil in the soap used to clean the wool. Decanal also naturally occurs in almonds, apples, flowers, apricots, artichokes, and avocados. Nonyl aldehyde (nonanal) is found in various vegetables, and is used as a food additive.

Due to environmental absorption, other extremely low levels of compounds may also be present in any mattress that uses natural organic materials, such as cotton or wool. Typically, these outgas completely in a fairly short period of time (four to eight hours, or days).

Decanal and nonanal are both approved as food flavoring or additive agents. Although either can be an irritant in higher exposures, I do not believe that at the low levels present these chemicals pose a human health risk. Neither of these chemicals are classified as harmful to the environment.

The VOCs from the 39 chemicals identified in the typical innerspring/pillow-top mattress produced a total emission of 4,002 ug/unit-hr. By comparison, the OMI innerspring-style mattress produced total emissions of 39 ug/unit-hr, or 97.5 percent less VOC emissions for the same 24-hour period. Applying my *Avoidance or Substitution Rule*, if you prefer sleeping on a traditional padded innerspring-style mattress, selecting a mattress manufactured by OMI would significantly reduce your exposure to chemical outgassing.

Long-term, low-level outgassing from many of the chemicals used to create a conventional mattress may be responsible for a variety of individual illnesses and symptoms, even though their outgassing levels may be well below what OSHA and the EPA consider to be harmful. That's because each of us has a unique chemical exposure threshold that is influenced by several conditions, one of which is the existing body burden of chemicals we are already carrying. Also, a person's immune system may already be compromised; his or her DNA may create a predisposition to specific chemicals that can cause hypersensitivity to certain chemicals; and/or daily exposure to other chemicals can create a synergistic reaction.

Chapter Four

Your Chemical Bedroom

"A good laugh and a long sleep are the best cures in the doctor's book."
—Irish Proverb

CONSUMERS ARE GROWING more and more sensitive to the vast array of chemicals used in the manufacture of the everyday items that are brought into their homes, and more specifically, into their bedrooms—the room in the home where people generally spend the most time and, therefore, has the highest potential for chemical exposure. I believe that health reactions to bedroom contaminants or pollutants go mostly unrecognized by the majority of us, and health symptoms are all too often ignored or blamed on other bacterial and viral causes.

Most Americans are trained from an early age to seek out a doctor, and then usually a drug, to take away headaches, sore throats, rashes, respiratory distress, and many other common ailments. We are not trained to suspect or seek out an environmental culprit in our home that could be causing the reaction or symptom.

Chem-tox.com makes it apparent that the cause of many of the above health conditions can in fact be a new mattress, rather than bacteria or viruses.

And it is not just the toxins and allergens in a typical new mattress that we need to be concerned with. Other products in and around the bedroom can also make it a potentially hazardous sleep zone.

In this chapter we will briefly explore the chemical impacts of products that are closely associated with mattresses, as well as products in and adjacent to our sleeping space, such as bathrooms and closets.

The Chemicals in Your Bed Linens

What is the "smell of clean" to you? Is it odorless, or is it the fragrances we have all grown to relate to as clean, but which are in fact residues from the chemicals used to manufacture, launder and clean everyday products?

Sheets, blankets, and pillows are all capable of giving off toxic VOCs. They are made with petroleum-based fibers and cotton grown with pesticides, herbicides, and defoliants. The yarns are treated with chemicals to make them fire retardant and wrinkle resistant. Many fiber-finishing processes incorporate formaldehyde (used to reduce wrinkling) directly into yarns to ensure that the chemical treatment will survive many washings.

One of the questions I am frequently asked is, "Which chemicals remain in sheets and bedding after they have been laundered?" Unfortunately, no study has been published that sets up a baseline for bed linen VOCs and then evaluates it after a certain number of washings under controlled conditions. Also, laundry products themselves can add undesirable chemicals to sheets and bedding.

What Chemicals Do You Launder into Your Sheets?

Did you ever wonder why laundry products incorporate language such as "Warning," "Danger," and "Caution" as part of their labels? The EPA advises consumers to be aware that laundry products contain cleaning agents (chemicals) that may irritate skin or make consumers more sensitive to other chemicals.

Here are a few of the "main offenders":

Surfactants: Chemicals such as alkyl benzene sulfonates (ABS) and linear alkyl benzene sulfonates (LAS), often referred to as "anionic surfactants" on labels, are designed to help water penetrate fabrics. They are known to cause allergic reactions such as skin rashes. Diethanolamines, triethanolamine, and monoethanolamine are also used as surfactants. These are generally slow to biodegrade, and react with elements in the atmosphere to form nitrosames, generally accepted to be potent carcinogens. Alkyl ammonium chloride—also used as a surfactant—releases formaldehyde, a known toxin and recognized carcinogen.

Optical brighteners are designed to trick your eye into believing that "whites are whiter." They are deadly to fish, and may cause skin reactions.

Petroleum distillates or (naphthas) on a label can mean just about any synthetic chemical that can be extracted from oil. Because of the broad number of chemical possibilities, I cannot comment on their risks, but do know that I don't want to sleep with them.

Polycarboxylates and **EDTA** (ethylene diamino tetra acetate) are added to laundry products to replace the phosphates that caused so much aquatic havoc in years past. Although they are considered safer than phosphates, they do not biodegrade, and are petroleum based.

Artificial fragrances are added to just about every commercial laundry and cleaning product, and current laws do not require that manufacturers list the specific ingredients. So again, it is not possible to comment specifically on, or for consumers to evaluate precisely, the risks these fragrances pose.

A single artificial fragrance can contain literally hundreds of different chemicals.

It is commonly known in the fragrance industry that ingredients such as camphor, ethanol, diethyl phthalate (DEP), dimethyl phthalate (DMP), and many of the 3,000 other chemicals enumerated on the list of fragrance chemicals published by the Research Institute for Fragrance Materials, are suspected endocrine disruptors, irritants, and carcinogens. A study done by the University of California, San Diego, also found that irritations and reactions can continue after the scent itself is no longer discernable, which makes it difficult for consumers to directly associate cause and effect with a particular event or product. Ingredients in artificial fragrances can cause headaches, nausea, shortness of breath, muscle weakness, and central nervous system depression.

The Consumer Product Safety Commission (CPSC) can stop the sale of any product it considers toxic or dangerous to consumers. However, in its evaluations, the CPSC does not regulate any of the specific ingredients included in the category of "artificial fragrance." No agency regulates the expression "fragrance-free," and the FDA regulates only fragrances that are considered to be cosmetics. Since most fragrances are made from non-dissolving petroleum, it is no surprise that they are found in waterways throughout the United States.

Fabric Softeners

Fabric softeners use chemicals to modify a fabric's surface. Some leave a film on the surface of fibers, while others are absorbed by the fibers, causing colors to dull. The EPA has found the following chemicals contained in fabric softeners: alpha-terpinol, benzyl alcohol, benzyl acetate, camphor, chloroform, ethyl acetate, limonene, linalol, pentane, and who knows what other chemicals in the artificial fragrances that are added to cover up the smell of other chemicals. In addition, quaternary ammonium compounds are frequently part of fabric softener formulas.

These chemicals have been linked to central nervous system disorders, cancer, respiratory tract irritation, and symptoms such as headache, nausea, dizziness, skin rash, and allergic reactions. Why would anyone want these chemicals in his or her bedroom?

Pre-Spotters/Stain Removers

The next time you are at the supermarket, find these products and read the labels. It will be a fast read, because manufacturers are not required to list the ingredients. At the most, you will find a mention of artificial fragrances or surfactants. Here are just a few of the typical chemicals used in these kinds of products: sodium dodecylbenzene sulfonate, urea, petroleum distillates, proteolytic enzymes, triethanolamine, and dipropylene glycol methyl.

So how does a consumer evaluate such products for potential chemical exposure? With great difficulty. My solution is simply to follow the **Avoidance or Substitution Rule**: Find a product in a health food store that lists all its ingredients, make your own, or live with the stains on your clothes. There are a number of books and websites that offer home recipes for most common laundry and cleaning products.

Chlorine Bleach

The EPA classifies chlorine as a pesticide, stating that its sole purpose is to kill living organisms. Chlorine, when combined with water and other natural compounds, forms trihalomethanes (THMs). THMs in turn trigger the production of free radicals in the body, which can be responsible for cell damage and are considered highly carcinogenic. The Environmental Defense Fund has stated that, "Although concentrations of these carcinogens (THMs) are low, it is precisely low levels that cancer scientists believe are responsible for the majority of human cancers in the United States."

TIPS to Make Your Linens Safer

Buy products made from 100 percent certified organic cotton rather than petroleum-based fabrics such as polyester.

Avoid products that claim to be "100 percent natural cotton," "Undyed and Unbleached Cotton," or "Green Cotton." These marketing expressions mean absolutely nothing, as they all describe cotton grown with pesticides.

Stay away from fabrics with any form of stain treatment or wrinkle resistance.

Instead of using a chemical fabric softener, try adding a quarter cup of baking soda to the wash cycle or half a cup of white vinegar to the rinse cycle.

Use a non-chlorine hydrogen-peroxide bleach.

Check out the ingredients in the laundry products at your local health food store.

Avoid products that do not disclose their ingredients.

Toxins in Your Bedroom Furniture

Inside your home, formaldehyde is frequently outgassed from the wood products used to construct bedroom furniture. Particleboard, fiberboard, and plywood (chipboard or OSB) are made using adhesives that contain urea-formaldehyde or phenol-formaldehyde resin.

In addition, veneers are applied with a variety of chemical adhesives and then finished with wood stains and surface sealers. Oil stains that utilize mineral spirits as a solvent are unhealthful for consumers and contaminate our water supply. Rags soaked in it can even instantaneously combust. Surface coatings that use toxic ingredients such as polyurethane are produced through condensation and a chemical reaction of diisocyanate and a polyol, with hydroxybenzotriazole or other antioxidation chemicals. The end result is a host of potentially carcinogenic and irritating chemicals that you don't want to breathe all night.

TIPS for Choosing Safer Bedroom Furniture

- Try to purchase furniture made from solid wood (preferably other than pine), rather than pressed-wood products.
- Seek out furniture that has been finished with water-based solvents, as opposed to traditional oil-based stains and urethane finishes.

Toxins Under Your Bed (Dust)

We all learn from an early age that dust bunnies live under beds. Today, many people do not consider these clumps of fuzz so benign.

Many books and articles have been written about the biological and chemical contaminants found in dust, and how exposure to them can have both short-term and long-term health effects. My focus in this book is simply to make you aware of how that can be affecting your sleeping environment.

Today many mattresses are used without a traditional box-spring foundation, the mattress instead being placed directly upon a wood-slat platform bed. This raises several "dust concerns."

When people dust or vacuum under their beds, or when air currents disturb the area under a bed, the dust rises, and a percentage of its contaminants adhere to the fabric on the bottom of the mattress. When the mattress is flipped, the dust layer is then positioned next to the sleeper's face.

The Paint on Your Walls

Anyone who has ever walked into a freshly painted room can smell the irritating odors, fumes, or offgassing. Have you ever wondered what

> ## TIPS for Minimizing the Effects of Under-Bed Dust
> • Thoroughly vacuum the surface of a flipped mattress before sleeping on it.
> • Use an underbed pad to protect the bottom of the mattress—not just from dust, but also from abrasive damage caused by the mattress rubbing against the wood surface of the platform bed.

causes this pungent odor? The reason you can smell paint when it is wet, but not dry, is because ingredients in liquid paint, such as oil-based derivatives and solvents, evaporate into the air as the paint dries. In other words, the toxins within the paint are released as gases into the air. And just because paint dries and changes from a liquid to a solid does not mean that the toxins have disappeared.

In a scientific chamber-emission study by J. Chang, L. E. Sparks, Z. Guo, and R. Fortmann, published in the March 1999 issue of the *International Journal of Indoor Environment and Health*, samples of latex paint were analyzed for emissions of VOCs. Four VOCs were found to be present: propylene glycol, ethylene glycol, 2-(2-butoxyethoxy) ethanol (BEE), and texanol.

Ethylene glycol, while great for coating surfaces, has long been suspected of damaging health effects. Glycols have been federally classified as toxic air contaminants or hazardous pollutants since 1993. Low-level exposures have been associated with upper respiratory tract irritation, conjunctivitis, and temporary corneal clouding. The State of California has determined, under Proposition 65, that ethylene glycol is a male reproductive and developmental toxicant. The same study indicated that its outgassing could last as long as 200 days. In addition, VOCs from paint can include such toxic gases as benzene and vinyl chloride.

Different paint products such as epoxy urea-formaldehyde, latex, and oil-based paints use different ingredients. The carrier in oil-based paints is composed entirely of unhealthful VOCs, ranging from 250 to 800 grams/liter (g/l). Most latex paints contain between 0 and 200 g/l of VOCs. The EPA established VOC guidelines for paints that took effect in

September 1999, stating that it cannot contain greater than 250 g/l, and 380 g/l in non-flat paint. The reduction of VOC levels is aimed at reducing ground-level ozone levels.

The EPA estimates that offgassing from architectural coatings accounts for about 9 percent of VOC emissions from all consumer and commercial products. These fumes become an even more serious issue when they are present in confined indoor spaces such as the home.

In addition to VOCs, chemicals called biocides are also added to latex paint, acting as preservatives and fungicides. Biocides found in paint include copper, arsenic disulfide, phenol, formaldehyde, and quaternary ammonium compounds. The EPA has shown that formulations with formaldehyde can offgas, despite manufacturer claims.

While non- or low-VOC paint is the more healthful paint choice for everyone, it is even more important for people with allergies, asthma, or chemical sensitivities. Using a product with the lowest possible VOC content will yield the lowest overall health risk. It is nearly impossible to eliminate VOCs in paint. However, using the EPA's Reference Test Method 24, any paint with VOCs in the range of 5 g/l or less can be called "Zero VOC." Also, remember that the health effects associated with paint will diminish significantly as it dries. The best thing you can do is create conditions inside your home that encourage rapid drying of the paint, and ventilate odors out of the house as rapidly as possible.

California was the first state to enact laws limiting VOC content in paints and coatings. New York, New Jersey, Texas, and Arizona followed shortly thereafter with laws of their own.

TIPS for Making Your Bedroom Walls Safer

- Read the labels on all products, and select plant-based formulas whenever possible.
- Choose low- and no-VOC paints.
- If you must use paint that contains VOCs, select a latex paint with VOCs no higher than 250 g/1, or 380 g/1 for oil-based products.
- As a general rule when you paint or stain, keep the windows open. (I personally keep a window open slightly for a year after I have painted or stained an area.)

Your Floor: Carpets and Cleaners

Carpet Flooring

Once reserved for the wealthy, carpets and rugs have become common-place in the American home. According to the Carpet and Rug Institute, 2.3 billion square yards of carpet were produced in 2004 in the United States alone. This is an increase of over 70 percent since the 1950s.

Like many other household products and furnishings, new carpeting can be a source of chemical emissions and an ideal environment for allergens and dust mites. Carpets and the products that typically accompany their installation, such as adhesives and sealants, emit VOCs. Modern carpeting is overwhelmingly made from petroleum-based synthetic fibers such as nylon, olefins, and polyester. These fibers are made from chemical ingredients that are derived from natural gas and petroleum. The fibers are further treated with a variety of chemicals to achieve stain protection and fire resistance. They are then treated with more chemical fungicides and pesticides. The tufted carpet is then attached to a backing (made mainly of polypropylene) using synthetic rubber, polyurethane, polyvinyl chloride, or ethylene vinyl acetate.

Typical synthetic carpeting has been found to outgas chemicals such as acetonitrile, azulene, benzene, diphenyl ethers, dodecane, tetrachloroethylene, toluene, xylene, ethylbenzene, and formaldehyde. These chemicals are associated with symptoms such as eye, nose, and throat irritation; headaches; skin irritations; shortness of breath or cough; and fatigue.

In 1988, the installation of new carpeting at EPA headquarters in Washington, D.C., led to a slew of complaints and health problems from the staff. This incident became the first highly publicized case of what is now typically referred to as "sick building syndrome." According to the EPA, this is used to describe "situations in which building occupants experience acute health and comfort effects that appear to be linked to time spent in a building, but no specific illness or cause can be identified."

In the EPA's case, the cause of the problem was never specifically verified, but speculation focused on the adhesives used to install the carpet and on a chemical by-product known as 4-PC (4-phenylcyclohexene), which was released from the carpet's backing material.

In 1992, studies were performed at an independent toxicology laboratory in which mice were exposed to air drawn from carpet samples that people suspected were making them sick. The mice displayed symptoms such as irritation of the eyes, nose, and throat; labored breathing; tremor; paralysis of the legs; and convulsions. Some of the mice in the study died as a result of exposure to carpet fumes. The researchers concluded that certain carpets release toxic chemicals into the air. (Interestingly, the researchers weren't testing just new carpeting—some of the samples were up to 12 years old.)

The results of this study, in addition to several hundred complaints associated with new-carpet installation, led the Consumer Product Safety Commission (CPSC) to study chemical emissions from carpets and the health effects associated with these emissions. Their study identified at least 30 chemicals released from carpets.

Of these chemicals, styrene and 4-PC (4-phenylcyclohexene) are the most notable. Both originate from the synthetic latex backing that is used on the majority of carpets. Styrene is a known toxin and suspected carcinogen, and while no studies have yet identified 4-PC as a toxic chemical, it has a very strong odor, even in small amounts. It is the chemical most responsible for the distinctive smell associated with new carpets. It is also less immediately volatile than many of the other chemicals measured, so it continues to be emitted at measurable levels for a longer period of time.

Yet despite the presence of these dangerous chemicals, the CPSC study found that chemicals emitted from carpeting are present at levels below those likely to contribute to adverse health effects. The number of health complaints associated with carpets continues to escalate.

Some researchers have suggested that two or more of the many chemicals emitted from a carpet may interact to cause a greater impact than that of any one substance. Another possible reason for the discrepancy is that the CPSC study tested four random samples, and it is likely that there are significant variations in chemical emanations from one carpet batch to the next. Thus, some batches may produce carpets with much higher emission levels than those tested in the CPSC study.

One component of the problem appears to be that some people are simply much more sensitized than others to the effects of chemicals.

These individuals with multiple chemical sensitivities (MCS) or environmental illness (EI) appear to be severely affected by conditions that most people consider normal. Advocates for the MCS and EI community point out that most members can identify a specific event when they were exposed to unusual levels of toxins that "tipped them over the edge." They warn that the syndrome may result from the cumulative effects of low-level chemical exposure, and that everyone is potentially at risk. In 1992, the Carpet and Rug Institute began a voluntary testing and labeling program through which each carpet line is tested four times a year for four categories of emissions: total VOCs, styrene, 4-PC, and formaldehyde. Maximum emission levels, measured at 24 hours after manufacture, are established as noted in Table 4.

Products that pass the test may carry a so-called "Green Label." This labeling system is clearly an improvement, as consumers are at least made aware of some of the chemicals used in the carpet-manufacturing process. However, this testing system is not without flaws. For starters, carpet testing is done only four times per year. This is not frequently enough to catch bad batches of carpet that crop up. In addition, the tests are checking far too few substances. For the past several years, the states of California and Washington have been pressing the industry to establish maximum emission standards that are stricter than the industry's current voluntary standards.

Table 4: Maximum Allowable Emission Criteria

Toxin	Maximum Allowable Emission (measured in mg/m^2)
Total Volatile Compounds	0.5
4-PC (4-Phenylcyclohexene)	0.5
Formaldehyde	0.05
Styrene	0.4

The carpet industry seems to focus on the premise that carpets only offgas during their initial installation. According to many health experts, however, older carpets may be just as bad or worse than new carpets. Once a carpet is installed, it acts like a sink for anything in the air, trapping particulates and pollutants. Pollutants such as pesticides or particulate matter that are tracked inside on shoes or wheels can also become lodged in the fibers of a carpet. When these pollutants are present outdoors, they are eventually broken down by ultraviolet light from the sun. Once they become trapped in indoor carpeting, however, nothing can remove them. They become absorbed into the carpet, where they are stored and eventually released into the air. (By the way, if you are thinking of getting your bedroom carpets cleaned to rid yourself of accumulated industrial chemicals, keep in mind that carpet-cleaning companies often use solvents that themselves contain ingredients such as glycol ethers and other toxic chemicals.) Wool fibers, because they are more absorbent, appear to have an even greater capacity than synthetics for trapping contaminants such as formaldehyde and nitrogen oxides.

Finally, it is important to note that carpeting itself is not the only product that can negatively affect indoor air quality. Even the carpet industry is quick to point out that carpet adhesives and sealants produce far more airborne pollutants than do carpets, especially in the first few weeks. Other products that may affect indoor air quality include carpet backing and pads.

TIPS for Making Your Carpet Safer

- If you already have carpeting, be sure to thoroughly vacuum it several times a week to reduce trapped pollutants.
- If you are considering a new carpet purchase, check the label to find carpeting with the lowest possible toxic emissions. Also, ask your installer to use low-emission adhesives and sealants during installation.
- Ask the dealer to air out the carpeting in a clean, well-ventilated room for several days prior to delivery. Be sure you will have adequate ventilation while it is being installed and for several weeks after.

Wood Flooring and Cleaners

Almost all wood and wood-based flooring contains formaldehyde, which can be emitted into the air after installation. In a recent study of formaldehyde emissions in the home, Thomas J. Kelly of the Battelle Memorial Institute in Columbus, Ohio, and his colleagues tested 55 household products, from wrinkle-free shirts to latex paint. They placed each product in a closet-sized monitoring chamber for 24 hours and measured the formaldehyde in the air. An acid-cured wood-floor finish—a product that gives wood floors a high-gloss shine—was the worst offender in the study. As mentioned earlier, formaldehyde is a known carcinogen that can also cause a number of acute symptoms such as irritation to the eyes, nose, and throat; difficulty breathing; and headache.

Another issue of concern regarding wood flooring is the cleaners and waxes that are used to care for it. Most household wood cleaners and polishes are made from petrochemical solvents that add to the level of toxins in our indoor air. Nitrobenzene is one such chemical that is frequently used in wood cleaners and polishes. This chemical can cause skin discoloration, shallow breathing, vomiting, and death. It is also associated with cancer and birth defects. For a natural alternative to commercial wood-care products, mix 1/2 cup vinegar and 1/2 cup vegetable oil. Rub on floor and buff with a clean, dry cloth.

TIPS for Making Your Bedroom Floors Safer

- If you can choose your floor covering, go with a traditional hard wood or newer eco-flooring alternatives, such as cork, bamboo, or sisal, which are usually finished with a nontoxic surface coating.
- Instead of carpet, choose loose area rugs made from natural fibers such as wool, silk, or cotton.
- If you must have carpet, choose water-based adhesives and other "green" alternatives for installation.
- Remember to air out the room as much as possible after your new floor is installed.

What's Coming Out of Your Closet?

There are over 30,000 dry-cleaning facilities in the United States. Unfortunately, 95 percent of these facilities use the toxic chemical perchloroethylene as their primary cleaning solvent. What we call "dry cleaning" is not actually dry at all. Rather, your clothing is soaked in perchloroethylene, also known as "perc," and tetrachloroethylene. Perc is a colorless, nonflammable liquid that is very hazardous to human health. This persistent toxic chemical is highly volatile and has been linked to cancer, birth defects, damage to the central nervous system, and a host of short-term effects such as dizziness, nausea, and shortness of breath.

The National Institute of Environmental Health Sciences states that "Short-term exposure to perc can cause adverse health effects on the nervous system that include dizziness, fatigue, headache, sweating, inco-ordination, and unconsciousness. Long-term exposure can cause liver and kidney damage." The International Agency for Research on Cancer classifies perc as a probable carcinogen.

While perc is supposed to evaporate while clothes are at the dry cleaner's, it is often trapped by the plastic bags that wrap the garments. This toxic chemical can then outgas for up to a week after you bring your clothes home. Even greater threats are posed to people working at dry-cleaning establishments and those who live nearby.

Your best bet for avoiding perc is to steer clear of dry cleaners alto-gether. The EPA is encouraging dry cleaners to voluntarily phase out perc. If you must dry-clean your clothes and your cleaner uses perc, be sure to take the plastic bags off your clothes and let them air on a clothes-line or in a closet away from your bedroom if possible until the telltale "sweet" smell is gone.

When we built our home, we created a closet off the living room specifically to hang our "fresh" dry cleaning in so it could outgas before

TIPS for Making Your Closet Air Fresher

- Choose a dry cleaner that uses "wet cleaning" technology without perchloroethylene.
- Allow cleaned clothes to air out in fresh air before putting them in your closet.
- Keep clothes in a separate area away from your bedroom, with the plastic removed, for at least a week before moving them closer to your sleeping area.
- Avoid mothballs, as they can outgas 1,4-dichlorobenzene (para-DCCB), which is listed by the California Department of Health Services as a known human carcinogen.

we brought it into the walk-in closet off our bedroom, and it has worked out very well.

Another option is to look for a dry cleaner that uses "wet cleaning" technology. In the last several years, "wet cleaning" has been developed to clean clothes that need delicate handling. It allows the cleaning agency to spend less money on equipment and chemicals, and more on training store personnel to use a combination of hand washing, spot cleaning, steaming, and pressing to clean delicate garments. "Wet cleaners" use specialized washing machines that clean delicate fabrics without stressing them, and the cleaning agents used at such facilities are purchased with an eye toward protecting both environmental and human health.

Electronics in Your Bedroom

We live in a world in which we are literally surrounded by different forms of invisible electrical influences. Each of us sleeps in his or her own unique environment of electromagnetic fields generated from both natural and human-made electrical sources. These electromagnetic fields are referred to as "EMFs," or more specifically, extremely low frequency (ELF) and very low frequency (VLF) fields. EMFs have a spectrum of frequencies ranging from X-rays (1 billion hertz) down to the electrical wiring in most homes (60 hertz).

The earth itself produces static fields of electromagnetism, which are thought to be produced by electric currents flowing deep within the planet's core. The earth's electromagnetic field pulses at about eight hertz (Hz). This is about the same pulse level as that of human bioelectrical functions, such as the electric signals that cross cell membranes and control actions within the nervous and endocrine systems. Our natural environment also produces electric fields through air turbulence and atmospheric activity such as lightning.

In addition to these naturally occurring sources, artificial electromagnetic fields are created whenever power is generated, transmitted, or used. Electricity for your clock radio, electric blanket, heated waterbed, bedside lamp, television, remote control, electrical wiring, telephone, or computer all generate electric and magnetic fields surrounding your bed.

Some people believe that EMFs can disrupt normal electrical signals within the human body. These signals cross cell membranes and affect normal biological actions, chemical activity, and hormonal secretions. Others believe that EMFs can interfere with the body's natural defense mechanisms that are designed to respond to the damaging free radicals that are associated with conditions such as premature aging, skin disease, and cancer.

There is a great deal of debate over the cause-and-effect relationship between human health and EMFs. However, tests on animals exposed to typical household levels of electromagnetic fields (i.e., 60 Hz) found that the animals' nervous and hormonal systems were negatively influenced. Studies on animal cell and tissue cultures indicated that basic cell activity is affected by low-frequency fields.

In February 2004, researchers Henry Lai and Narendra Singh of the University of Washington's Department of Bioengineering concluded that when rats were exposed to a low-level, 60-Hz magnetic field for 24 hours, breaks in brain-cell DNA strands and other serious brain-cell damage occurred. Previous to this study, scientists had maintained that EMF fields were not strong enough to break the chemical bonds in a living organism.

The health risks associated with EMFs are influenced by the specific strength of the field, the length of exposure, and each person's individual threshold or particular sensitivity to magnetic influences. It has been suggested that EMFs may be linked to health effects such as leukemia, brain tumors, and breast cancer. Scientists and health experts are currently divided on the risks involved with exposure to ELF and VLF magnetic fields. However, a workshop held by the World Health Organization (WHO) in 2004 concluded that:

"... scientific research can provide some measure of confidence that short-term, acute exposures up to about 1-2 T [1000-2000 milliT] should be safe ... However, it is not possible to determine whether there are any long-term health consequences even from exposure in the milliT range because, to date, there are no well-conducted epidemiological studies with sufficient power to be able to come to any conclusion on this, and there are no good long-term animal studies."

In the bedroom we spend hours surrounded by products that produce EMFs, such as clocks, radios, reading lamps, telephones, televisions, and computers. These fields continually pulse through our bodies during our sleeping hours.

Electric blankets are another significant source of EMFs. Some electric blankets generate a field in excess of 20 mG (milligauss) or more. Standing in front of a microwave exposes you to about 10 mG. Newer electric blankets are often promoted as "Low-EMF" products. These blankets typically generate a field within the 5 to 10 mG range. Electric blankets and waterbed heaters are of particular concern because they are used in such close proximity to the body, exposing the sleeper to relatively high magnetic fields for an extended period of time each night.

In addition, synthetic fabrics can also generate an electrostatic charge. Each of us has experienced an electric discharge or "shock" after walking across a synthetic carpet and touching a grounded object. We have also experienced the electrostatic charges that build up on synthetic fibers, causing "static cling." Many people believe that sleeping within a synthetic-fabric environment surrounds the body in a low-level electrostatic charge that may disrupt its natural biological balance.

TIPS for Avoiding EMF Exposure

There are better ways to avoid EMF exposure. Professor M. Granger Morgan of Carnegie-Mellon University coined the term "prudent avoidance" to describe the simple solution of limiting your exposure time and increasing your distance from EMF sources. Here are a few ideas:

- Move electronics in your bedroom so that they are further away from your body. For example: If the clock in your bedroom is powered by an electric motor, it can be a significant source of EMFs. Instead of keeping it near your head on your nightstand, increase your distance by moving it to a piece of furniture on the other side of the room, or replace it with one that uses batteries.
- Place other sources of EMFs, such as electric space heaters, electric baseboard heaters, floor fans, air-conditioning units, and telephones, as far away from the bed as possible.
- Keep in mind that EMFs pass through walls. Televisions generate magnetic fields in all directions, and computers emit these fields mostly from the rear and sides. For this reason, don't place your baby's crib—or any bed—on a wall directly behind these products.

Finally, there is a prominent theory among naturalists that the inner-springs in a modern mattress can become magnetized by a room's wiring and electrical products. Once magnetized, the metal innersprings can generate their own direct-current (DC) magnetic field, which may disrupt sleeping patterns and interfere with the body's natural bioelectrical processes. Years ago, I attended a show in Europe where a Bau-Biologist (building biologist) held a magnet over an innerspring mattress that had been in a home for five years. When she held a compass over the bed, I was surprised to see the compass needle deflect from the true polar readings. I have often thought of that experience, and have slept on an organic natural rubber mattress ever since.

There are several ways to minimize your exposure to EMFs in your bedroom. Some companies sell magnetic mattress pads as a method for counteracting the magnetic fields generated from innersprings. The premise behind these products is that the body can be shielded from electrical stress by laying a protective magnetic sheet under the mattress to focus, ground, or diffuse the magnetic influence of the innersprings.

Bathroom Adjacent to the Bedroom

Many homes have a bathroom next to the bedroom, and the occupants have probably never considered that the air from that room can easily mingle with and contaminate their bedroom.

Have you ever taken a look at the ingredients in your bathroom products? It's not just the cleaning products that are suspect. What chemicals are in that deodorizer plugged into the electric outlet? And don't forget the aerosol hair spray, deodorant, and other personal-care products.

Bathroom Products That
Can Contaminate Your Bedroom

Although far from a complete list, here are some of the worst products that can compromise bedroom air quality:

Toilet-Bowl Cleaners and Deodorizers

The highly caustic chemicals used in these products actually produce toxic gases, such as hydrochloric acid, which is a respiratory irritant. Often made with 1,4-dichlorobenzene (a pesticide known to be carcinogenic) and ammonium chloride (a chemical corrosive), it doesn't belong in your home at all, let alone in your bedroom's air.

Sink and Tile Cleaners

Breathing the vapors produced by these products—made from extremely caustic ingredients such as bleach and phosphoric acid—can actually burn your lung tissue. They may also contain ammonia and other chemicals recognized as carcinogens and reproductive toxins. I suggest you find a safer alternative rather than use these products in an area that can contaminate the air quality of your bedroom.

Mold and Mildew Cleaners

Most often sold as aerosol sprays, the fine mist created by products such as these can contain chemicals such as kerosene, formaldehyde, chlorine, phenols, and literally hundreds of other active ingredients. Although not created to be used in bedrooms, that is where much of their emissions wind up.

Air Fresheners and Deodorizers

These products, whether solid or aerosol, release nerve-deadening carcinogenic chemicals that are designed to coat nasal tissues with compounds whose sole purpose is to interfere with your sense of smell. The popular solid plug-in type actually breaks down chemicals into even smaller particles than do aerosol sprays. Both products create air contaminants that travel on indoor air currents into your bedroom if you permit it.

Personal-Care and Beauty Products That Can Contaminate Your Bedroom

Here are just a few of the products from this group that can cause the worst bedroom air contamination:

Nail-Polish Removers

Most of us can remember the odor associated with nail-polish removers. They contain acetone, which when inhaled can cause short-term symptoms such as light-headedness, headaches, confusion, nausea, and irritation of the respiratory system. Long-term exposure has been found to potentially damage the liver, kidneys, and nervous system. They have also been associated with birth defects. Such products are frequent bedroom air contaminants.

Hair Colorants and Permanents

Most hair colorants and home permanents contain VOCs such as formaldehyde and ammonia, in addition to their petroleum-based coal-tar derivatives. These chemicals will gladly hitch a ride on your indoor air currents and drift into your bedroom.

Hair Sprays and Styling Products

Often delivered through aerosol or pump sprays, these products produce fine droplets that become readily airborne. Many contain recognized hormone disruptors such as diethanolamine (DEA), monoethanolamine (MEA), and triethanolamine (TEA), as well as polyvinylpyrrolidone (PVP), which is actually a plasticizer. These chemicals can also combine with nitrates to form nitrosamines, which are known carcinogens. You don't want to breathe these chemicals in your bedroom.

Body Powders

The basic ingredient for this class of product is usually talc, which is a recognized carcinogen when inhaled. Such products produce a cloud of fragrance that should be kept out of sleeping environments.

A Note on the Ingredient "Fragrance"

You will find the ingredient "fragrance" in almost every product in your home, but you will be hard-pressed to evaluate its potential for exposing you and your family to unhealthy VOCs.

The FDA does not require any product using fragrance to disclose the chemicals they used to create the scent. The National Institute of Occupational Safety and Health (NIOSH) analyzed approximately 3,000 chemicals used in personal-care products and published the following results: 884 of the chemicals were toxic, 778 caused acute toxicity, 376 caused skin and eye irritations, 314 caused biological mutation, 218 caused reproductive complications and 146 caused tumors. There are literally thousands of fragrances that we know very little about, and their chemical ingredients are not required to be listed on product labels. Fragranced products can be as much as 95 percent petrochemically derived, and they are all capable of migrating into your sleeping quarters.

Of particular concern to the FDA and other health experts throughout the world is the "cocktail effect" that may occur when different chemicals are mixed in and on the body. While some products are tested for reactions such as skin irritations, there is little information published on potential effects from low-level, long-term exposures to specific products or their individual ingredients.

In 2005, the FDA finally issued an unprecedented warning to the cosmetics industry that it was time to inform consumers that most personal-care products have not been safety tested. Eighty-nine percent of the 10,500 some odd ingredients used in personal-care products have not been evaluated for safety by the FDA or the industry-appointed Cosmetic Ingredient Review Panel.

Cosmetic-industry spokespeople say that human exposure to individual substances and potential toxins falls far below the levels at which scientists test each substance in laboratory studies. However, no one is exposed to just a single dose of one particular chemical. Consumers, in practice, are exposed to any number of chemical combinations. A 2003 study conducted by the Centers for Disease Control and Prevention (CDC) found more than 116 different chemical compounds, including dioxins (by-products of chlorine that have been linked to cancer) and phthalates that impair our reproductive function, in a wide range of personal-care products used by a sample of both adults and children.

Bathroom Contaminants Can Come from Your Shower

According to an article in *New Scientist* magazine, breathing the air around a shower or bath increases your exposure to VOCs 6 to 100 times more than drinking the same water. When you take a hot shower or bath, the heat of the water makes the chlorine in the municipally treated tap water react to produce harmful VOCs. Often these VOCs drift from the bathroom into adjacent sleeping areas, where they become absorbed by linens and pillows.

A study published in *Environmental Health Perspectives* analyzed the breath of participants for compounds regulated in water supplies to determine the route of uptake from tap water. According to the study's authors, "traditional risk assessments for water often only consider ingestion exposure to toxic chemicals, even though showering has been shown to increase the body burden of certain chemicals due to inhalation exposure and dermal absorption." In other words, even if you filter your tap water before drinking it, contaminants are still entering your system through your skin and lungs while you shower. The longer the shower, the greater the concentration of chemicals you are exposed to. Many of these contaminants are known carcinogens.

Another study, performed by researchers at Brooks Air Force Base in Texas, characterized the emission rates of several chemicals in a full-size experimental shower. The study analyzed emissions of trichloroethylene and chloroform, two compounds that are considered highly volatile organic chemicals. In a typically hot shower (about 105°F) the rates of emission were 80 percent for trichloroethylene and 60 percent for chloroform. As you may expect, both of these chemicals are associated with a host of negative health risks.

Trichloroethylene is a colorless liquid that is used as a solvent for cleaning metal parts. According to the Agency for Toxic Substances and Disease Registry, "Breathing small amounts [of trichloroethylene] may cause headaches, lung irritation, dizziness, poor coordination, and difficulty concentrating. Breathing large amounts of trichloroethylene may cause impaired heart function, unconsciousness, and death."

Chloroform is a colorless liquid with a pleasant, nonirritating odor and a slightly sweet taste. In the past, chloroform was used as an inhaled anesthetic during surgery, but today it is more commonly used to make other chemicals. Chloroform can also be formed when chlorine is added to water. Breathing in chloroform can cause fatigue, dizziness, and headache. In the long term, breathing or ingesting chloroform may cause damage to your liver and kidneys.

It is important to realize that skin is the largest organ of your body. Whatever gets put on your skin potentially may be absorbed into your body, into your bloodstream, and into your organs. Essentially, whatever is toxic to put in your mouth is toxic on your skin, and if it contributes to the air quality in your bedroom, you are breathing it as well.

TIPS for Safer Bathrooms (and Cleaner Bedroom Air)

- Read product labels, and avoid those that contain words such as "caution," "hazardous," or "dangerous," as well as those that don't list their ingredients. There is an excellent Canadian website, www.lesstoxicguide.ca, that is a great source of safe alternative formulas for most home and personal-care products.
- Upgrade your bathroom exhaust fan, never clean any surface of the room without turning the fan on, and keep the door between the bathroom and bedroom closed as much as possible.
- If you have a window in the room, keep it open as much as possible. This will help draft air out of the bedroom area.
- Dyes and chemical treatments used on new bath towels can produce VOCs and be absorbed by your skin. Wash them at least five times before using, and preferably buy towels made from undyed, nonchemically grown or processed certified organic cotton.
- Have you ever smelled a vinyl shower curtain fresh out of its plastic package? Keep these VOCs out of your home by substituting a shower curtain made from certified organic cotton or hemp.
- Use a manual pump sprayer for personal-care products instead of high-VOC-producing pressurized aerosols.

Table 5: Toxins in Your Bedroom

Source	Toxins	Health Hazards
Mattresses and Linens	A "toxic soup" of chemicals such as pesticides, formaldehyde, PCBs, PBDEs, and boric acid	Symptoms such as headache, nausea, fatigue, and sore throat, as well as conditions such as allergic reaction, respiratory distress, reproductive dysfunction, and cancer
Laundry Detergents or Fabric Softener	Chlorine, petroleum distillates, phosphates, and benzyl acetate	Allergic reaction, immune-system suppression, and environmental damage—may also be linked to pancreatic cancer, and reproductive damage
Furniture	Formaldehyde	Cancer, irritation of the nose, throat, and skin, coughing, wheezing and nausea
Paint	Volatile Organic Compounds (VOCs)	Cancer, irritation of the eyes, nose, and skin, as well as headaches, nausea, convulsions, dizziness and nerve damage
Carpeting	VOCs, styrene, synthetic fibers, and dyes	Irritation of the eyes, nose, and throat, as well as more serious conditions such as cancer
Wood Floors	Formaldehyde	Known carcinogen
Dry-Cleaned Clothing	Perchloroethylene	Cancer, birth defects, damage to the central nervous system, and a host of short-term effects such as dizziness, nausea, and shortness of breath

Table 5: Toxins in Your Bedroom *continued*

Source	Toxins	Health Hazards
Electronics (clocks, computers, televisions, telephones, and electric blankets, etc.)	Electromagnetic fields (EMFs)	May affect normal biological actions, chemical activity, and hormonal secretions
Bathrooms	Chemicals in cleaning solutions and cosmetics	Cancer, upper respiratory distress, nausea, fatigue, headache, and allergic reaction

PART 2

The Information Void

CURRENTLY, THERE IS NO EFFECTIVE WAY for Americans to accurately assess the general level of chemicals and pollutants that they are exposed to on a daily basis. Nor do we know a great deal about the health consequences of these daily exposures or their short- and long-term environmental effects. Whose responsibility is it to help us evaluate the chemical contaminants present in our daily lives? How much of this responsibility falls on consumers, and what part should the government play in protecting the public?

The Politics of Chemicals and Public Health

"There is a time for many words, and there is also a time for sleep."
—Homer

OVER THE YEARS, a handful of exposure studies have been performed by agencies such as the Environmental Protection Agency, the Centers for Disease Control and Prevention, and the Environmental Working Group to determine what, where, and when pollutants come into contact with humans. The studies have shown that current federal and state regulations are failing to address many major indoor sources of pollutant exposure and their potential health risks. We are living in a time when the health risks from indoor air pollution produced by consumer products are far less regulated than the risks from the traditional factory pollution sources that contaminate outdoor air.

This "regulation gap" has led to an interesting paradox. We place our trust in environmental regulations to keep toxins out of our environment and our bodies, assuming that if a substance is not banned or under investigation, it must be safe. Yet the places and products we consider safest (our homes and the products with which we come into contact each day, such as our mattresses) can actually be our greatest sources of chemical exposure. The vast majority of consumer products are not tested for chemical-exposure risks, and when a product *is* tested, the information is not passed along to the consumer.

Much of this "information void" occurs because the majority of the chemicals we are exposed to on a daily basis entered the American product mainstream without adequate human or environmental toxicology studies in the first place. In fact, it wasn't until 1979 that the federal government passed the Toxic Substances Control Act, and even then, it only applied to *new* chemicals being used in consumer products. No provisions were made for retroactive testing or evaluations of chemicals introduced before 1979.

Of the roughly 100,000 chemicals now in common commercial use, only about 2 percent have ever been tested for carcinogenicity. It is no wonder that cancers are increasing at an alarming rate. In 1901, cancer was being diagnosed in about 1 in 8,000 Americans. Today, that figure is 1 in 3.

As exposure studies continue to show, we are affected by a wide range of non-food and non-pharmaceutical chemicals—chemicals that can cause adverse health effects and that are contained in common products that currently receive little or no pre-market testing in the United States. Health experts agree that humans can be harmed by any substance that is persistent, accumulative, carcinogenic, or toxic to any of the body's systems. Research has shown that toxins are showing up in all the wrong places (e.g., pesticides in human breast milk).

As consumers, we need to use the information we gather about toxins and our environment to make powerful choices with our wallets. We should promote the use and production of safer alternatives to common products and practices that pose unnecessary exposure risks. **For almost every toxic product that enters our home or our environment, there is a safer alternative that could provide the same function with less toxicity.** For example, we could choose personal-care products and laundry supplies without synthetic fragrances, paints and varnishes that are low in VOCs, and pest-control products based on integrated pest management rather than synthetic chemicals.

And as mentioned earlier, changing to an organic mattress is the easiest way to reduce chemical exposures in one-third of your life.

What Should Our Government Do?

One important step would be to require more extensive testing, labeling, and evaluation of products before they are allowed to enter the marketplace. Many people I have spoken with over the years have been under the impression that the Occupational Safety and Health Administration (OSHA) regulated such situations, but OSHA has never been concerned with consumer exposure to toxins within the home. They have always focused exclusively on workplace hazards. The organization most responsible at the federal level would be the Consumer Products Safety Commission, but they don't have the resources to address the issues of product emissions. Nor does the EPA have the legislative authority or staff to evaluate the personal safety of consumer products.

Since this book is mostly about mattresses, let's use that as our example. In our ideal world, a mattress law label—commonly referred to as the "Do Not Remove" label—would give the consumer the information he or she needs to determine the safety of that product. The law label would provide detailed information about the chemicals used to produce the raw materials present in the mattress, as well as any known health or environmental risks associated with short-term and long-term exposure. It would also list environmental consequences that occur when the product is disposed of.

Concerned? Get Active Politically

We need to become involved and ask our government representatives how such exposures occur, as well as how can they be prevented. Why are these pollutants being produced in the first place? The goal should be to phase them out and significantly reduce our reliance on them. To become more aware of the seriousness of the overall intrusion of chemicals into our lives and the consequences that result, I suggest you read *Synthetic Planet: Chemicals, Politics, and the Hazards of Modern Life* by Monica Casper (see suggested reading in Appendix 3).

The European Eco-Label Approach

In 1992, the European Union (EU) began supplementing its environmental laws with a voluntary Eco-label program for consumer products. This program is very specific in estimating the true personal and environmental risks associated with individual raw materials and their end products.

The goals of the Eco-label program are intended to promote the design, production, marketing, and use of products that have a reduced environmental impact during their life cycle, to provide consumers with better information on products' environmental impacts, and to help them make informed environmental choices in their purchases.

The Eco-label criteria take into account both the major environmental impact of a product and improvements that could be made to lessen that impact. These criteria are established by a board comprised of representatives from the European Commission, industry, consumers, environmentalists, and trade unions. This ensures transparency, scientific validity, and credible environmental protection. Products that pass designated environmental and performance standards may carry the Eco-label logo on their packaging. The label can be found on a wide variety of products, such as clothing, gardening products, household appliances, office equipment, and mattresses.

Before a product is eligible for the Eco-label logo, a complete Life Cycle Assessment is performed to analyze the following environmental impact categories:

- Effects on Global Warming
- Human Toxicity
- Contribution to Acid Rain
- Contribution to Ozone Depletion
- Eutrophication
- Smog Production
- Eco-Toxicity
- Landscape Demolition and Ecology
- Energy Usage
- Nuisance Factors
- Solid Waste

Here's a closer look at each of these categories and how the life cycle of a mattress may affect each of them:

Effects on Global Warming: This category has to do with the concern that the temperature of the earth's surface is rising at an accelerated rate as a direct result of human activity, which has altered the chemical composition of the atmosphere through the buildup of greenhouse gases—primarily carbon dioxide, methane, and nitrous oxide. The heat-trapping property of these gases is undisputed, although scientists and health experts continue to debate exactly how the earth's climate responds to them. Each of these greenhouse gases, particularly nitrous oxide and methane, can be emitted during the life cycle of a mattress. For example, gases are created in the production of the polyols used to make polyurethane foam, the styrene-butadiene used to make synthetic latex, and the polyethylene terephthalate used to make polyester. Carbon dioxide is also released when the mattress is incinerated.

Human Toxicity: The Eco-label program evaluates the toxicity of each substance used to make a mattress, together with the degradation and chronic toxicological effects of these substances.

Contribution to Acid Rain: During the production of the raw materials used to make most chemically laden mattresses, airborne emissions of acidic compounds may be released into the air. These emissions have the potential to contaminate water, soil, and living organisms.

Contribution to Ozone Depletion: Mattress raw materials and production processes use a number of halogen-containing gases or chlorofluorocarbons, as well as hydrogen chlorofluorocarbons. These substances contribute to the depletion of the earth's ozone layer.

Eutrophication: Runoff from certain chemical substances can significantly alter the chemical content of waterways. This can cause a process known as eutrophication, in which the growth of algae is stimulated and other aquatic life forms are starved of oxygen. During the manufacturing and production of a mattress, chemicals may be produced that contribute to eutrophication, such as phosphates, nitrogen, and potassium.

Smog Production: Smog is a kind of air pollution, originally named for the mixture of smoke and fog in the air. Today, "smog" describes a noxious mixture of air pollutants, including gases and fine particles that create a brownish-yellow or grayish-white haze. Smog is a concern in most major cities, but because it travels with the wind, it can affect sparsely populated areas as well. Smog is caused by the reaction between sunlight and chemical emissions such as VOCs and nitric oxides. These chemicals may also be released during the manufacturing of several mattress components, such as polyurethane, as well as from solvents used during the mattress manufacturing process.

Eco-Toxicity: Emissions and discharges of certain substances that are generated in the production and manufacturing of mattresses may adversely affect the environment. For example, mattresses that are awarded the Eco-label must not contain steel springs that are covered with a galvanic metallic layer, as this can create heavy-metal waste discharges that can be extremely damaging to the environment.

Landscape Demolition and Ecology: If you have ever seen a strip mine, you know the magnitude of the environmental damage that can be caused in the production of raw materials. The mining of minerals and fuels used to create a mattress can impact the natural landscape and the biodiversity of the environment.

Energy Usage: Under this criterion, a calculation is performed that analyzes all of the energy necessary to produce the raw materials and final product. For example, the energy used to create one kilogram of natural rubber is approximately 16 megajoules/kilogram. This can then be compared to the 100 megajoules/kilogram that is necessary to create the same amount of synthetic foam.

Nuisance Factor: This category analyzes the level of odor, noise, and other physical nuisances associated with the production of a mattress.

Solid Waste: The environmental impact of a product does not end once it is no longer useful. This category evaluates not only the durability of a mattress to ensure that it is long lasting, but also the ability of a mattress to biodegrade in a landfill and the toxicity of the waste products that would remain after a mattress is incinerated.

In conclusion, the Eco-label assures European mattress consumers that products exhibiting the label create a limited impact on air and water supplies during manufacturing, contain no ozone-depleting substances, contain minimal amounts of substances that may harm human and environmental health, have a reduced risk of causing allergic symptoms, and last as long as a non-ecological mattress.

It is a far cry from American mattress labels.

Mattress Flammability

MATTRESS FLAMMABILITY made headlines when new federal standards were implemented in July 2007 by the Consumer Products Safety Commission, and because of the research that has shown high levels of the fire retardant polybrominated diphenyl ether (PBDE) in breast milk. As the federal government adopts a more stringent open-flame test it forces mattress manufacturers to use chemical fire retardants and barriers to meet the standard. These chemicals, as a rule, have not been adequately tested for short- or long-term human toxicology. Nor is there any requirement to indicate which fire-retardant chemicals have been used in your mattress.

Mattress flammability is a two-edged sword. On one hand, all mattresses are highly combustible and produce toxic emissions when involved in a fire. On the other hand, the chemicals used to retard the flame may increase our toxic chemical exposures.

Let's look at the fire risk first. Mattress flammability standards were initially established in the 1970s in response to death and injuries caused by bedroom fires ignited by smoldering cigarettes. Current federal standards still use a lit cigarette as the ignition source when testing mattresses.

In March 2001, NBC's *Dateline* program performed a burn test on a conventional mattress. They dropped a match into a wastebasket next to the bed. Twenty seconds after the flames reached the mattress, it had ignited. Less than two minutes later, the mattress was in full flame and emitting cyanide and carbon monoxide. In less than three minutes, there was nothing left of the bed except steel springs and a burning pool of petroleum distillates (the primary derivatives of polyurethane foam and thermoplastic fibers, such as polyester, polypropylene, PVC, acrylic, and nylon). This is not surprising when you consider that many of the petrochemical-based components used to manufacture conventional mattresses have the same fire-combustibility rating as that of kerosene and gasoline.

But it is not just polyurethane foam and synthetic fibers that are combustible. All mattress components, with the exception of steel springs, are flammable under the right conditions. Fabric coverings, cellulose, synthetic battings, paddings and foams are all capable of ignition when a heat source is present with the right temperature and available oxygen. Some of these components burn faster than others, and some have different smoldering and smoke-producing characteristics. Thermoplastic fibers, such as polyester and nylon used in mattress covers, melt and shrink away from the fire source, actually exposing more of the mattress's other materials. In addition, as these fibers melt they can adhere to skin and clothing, making burns even worse.

In California, flammability standards have been increased even further, and the state now requires an open-flame test in addition to the burning cigarette test for mattresses.

Just How Flammable Are the Components in Your Mattress?

Covering Fabrics: As mentioned in earlier chapters, many different fibers can be used to produce the covering fabric for a mattress. Each has its own individual burn characteristics. For example, cotton produces high amounts of carbon monoxide when it is involved in low-oxygen smoldering conditions. When flame is involved, cotton produces carbon dioxide (a less-toxic gas). Nylon has just the opposite reaction, producing relatively nontoxic emissions at low temperatures and the highly toxic cyanide gas when flames are present. Wool, silk, and other nitrogen-based fibers can emit hydrogen cyanide. Wool tends to have the lowest contribution to smoke production, followed by cellulosic fibers, such as cotton, linen, and hemp. These fibers also tend to char in comparison to thermoplastic fibers, such as polyester, nylon, and polypropylene, which tend to melt. As they melt and shrink, these fibers can fall into the lower foam layers of the mattress or into the mattress core, where they can pool and continue to burn. Thermoplastic fibers also produce much more smoke than do natural fibers.

Battings: Wool batting is relatively resistant to ignition, and it has a natural tendency to self-extinguish. Cotton batting ignites far more easily, and has a tendency to smolder rather than burn. Battings made from either polyester or a cotton/polyester blend tend to generate higher heat, with polyester melting and igniting easier than all-cotton batting. Polyester batting is less flammable from heat sources such as a burning cigarette, but far more vulnerable to ignition when an open flame is present.

Core Materials: Flexible polyurethane foam is a highly flammable material. As mentioned earlier, some of the chemicals used to make polyurethane foam actually have the same combustion rating as kerosene and gasoline. It is a petroleum-based product with an open-celled structure that provides easy access to the oxygen that is necessary for combustion. In order for polyurethane foam to pass current flammability standards, it must be made with an array of flame-retardant chemicals. At low fire temperatures, flame-retardant polyurethane foam produces toxic gases such as volatile isocyanates and nonvolatile polyol. At higher temperatures, the polyol produces alkenes, alkynes, aldehydes, ketones, and finally black smoke. The isocyanates produce carbon monoxide and nitrogen-containing yellow smoke. As fire temperatures increase, this degrades to hydrogen cyanide and black smoke. The standard conventional mattress can contain between 50 to 100 pounds of polyurethane foam. When this foam is involved in a fire, it releases deadly poisonous gases at different temperature stages. Gases and gaseous compounds that can be emitted from burning polyurethane foam include two lethal gases—hydrogen cyanide and carbon monoxide—as well as toluene, benzene, acetaldehyde, butadiene, ethylene, ethane, propane, pyridine, benzonitrile, acetonitrile, acrylonitrile, methyl cyanobenzene, naphthalene, quinoline, indene, proprionitrile, and methyl pyridine.

Natural and synthetic latex have a lower ignition point than polyurethane foam, but also burn with a thick black smoke similar in appearance to burning tires. When rubber products burn, they can emit hydrogen sulphide, sulphur dioxide, carbon monoxide, carbon dioxide, and traces of acetic acid and other products.

Box Springs and Foundations: Conventional foundations are made from many of the same fabrics and paddings discussed earlier, as well as steel springs and wood. Wood requires a higher ignition temperature than do textiles. Once it does ignite, it can produce emissions such as acetic acid, aldehydes, carbon dioxide, carbon monoxide, ketones, methane, and tars. And although steel springs do not burn, they can add accelerants and smoke to the air if they are painted or treated with lubricants. At present, mattress flammability standards require the addition of an assortment of chemicals to reduce ignition potential. Fire-retardant chemicals are usually designed to reduce the heat or efficiency of combustion, but depending upon how they are incorporated into a material and the specific character-istics of the fire, some fire retardants can actually increase the production of carbon monoxide and smoke, and can add additional toxic chemicals to fire emissions. Furthermore, any carbon-based material can still burn, even with the addition of fire retardants and chemicals to its structure or surface.

Interliners, barrier layers, or fire blockers are also used between a mattress's covering fabric and padding layers to improve its flammability characteristics. These components may be made from flame-retardant cotton, polyester batting, glass fabrics, aluminized materials, flame-retardant foams, or even non-woven materials such as aramid. (Aramid is a non-flam-mable, dense material used in the production of bullet-proof vests.)

Changing Flammability Standards

California's flammability law (AB603) took effect in 2005, and is similar to the standards that took effect nationwide in July 2007. They require mattresses to have a significantly increased resistance to sources of open flames such as candles and matches. The "open-flame" test, as it has become known, is designed to simulate the heat and energy released from burning bedclothes. A dual-burner gas-flame device is used to apply flames to the sides and tops of the mattress and/or foundation. The test is conducted on complete mattress sets (for example, if a mattress is intended to be used with a box spring, the set will be tested together). The test consists of the following:

The side burner applies an open flame for 50 seconds, and simultaneously a top burner applies an open flame for 70 seconds. This "open flame" resembles a row of blow torches as opposed to a line of candles.

The mattress is observed for 30 minutes. A mattress fails the test if either:

- The total heat released by the mattress equals or exceeds 25 megajoules within 10 minutes of ignition;
- The peak heat released by the mattress equals or exceeds 200 kilowatts within the 30-minute test period.

The law initially attempted to regulate the flammability of a mattress for a 60-minute period, rather than a 30-minute period, bringing great debate from both industry and environmental experts. According to the Congressional testimony of David Orders, who spoke on behalf of the International Sleep Products Association: "The industry is concerned that meeting a 60-minute standard might inadvertently create more problems than it purports to solve. To meet a 60-minute requirement might force producers to use combinations of exotic materials that have never been used to make mattresses. How those materials will interact with each other is often unknown."

What's worse is that the proponents of this chemical flame-proofing standard are also looking into developing laws regarding the flammability of bed linens. This will require the application of similar fire-retarding chemicals to mattress pads, sheets, blankets, comforters, and pillows. When I provided testimony at the California TB 603 flammability hearings conducted by the California Bureau of Home Furnishing and Thermal Insulation, I raised the concern that while they were focusing on preventing the several hundred annual deaths attributed to mattress fires nationally, they should also consider the health effects associated with the potential chemical fire retardants that could be used to meet their flammability standard and that could expose millions of Americans to undetermined and undisclosed chemical risks. I received a response back that said that it was not their responsibility to assess the health effects of chemicals used to achieve fire standards. Here is a quote from their response to my objection:

"…Current worker safety and environmental laws in the United States address worker and consumer exposure to chemicals. No chemical may enter the U.S. market without extensive assessment and testing."

If only that were true. U.S. labeling laws do not currently require mattress retailers, manufacturers, or raw-material suppliers to pass flammability, environmental, or chemical disclosures on to the consumer.

The Consumer Product Safety Commission lists the following chemicals as the primary substances that can be applied to a mattress to meet this law:

- Boric Acid
- Formaldehyde
- Decabromodiphenyl Oxide
- Polybrominated Diphenyl Ethers (PBDEs)
- Antimony Trioxide
- Vinylidene Chloride
- Zinc Borate
- Melamine

These chemicals have never been studied for their long-term effects on humans when used in mattresses. They are likely to offgas for several years after application, but again, there are no studies to prove or disprove this fact. Unfortunately, without the appropriate data, the Consumer Product Safety Commission cannot make a quantitative risk analysis regarding the safety of these chemicals in our mattresses.

Flammability and Organic Mattresses

Organic mattresses pass all state and federal flammability standards primarily by using wool underneath the quilted top cover fabric. Wool is a natural fire retardant and it is not necessary to use any chemical fire retardants on the product.

Because of the extremely dangerous toxins produced by burning mattresses, I personally support the use of a single layer of a silica/cotton fabric inside an organic mattress. While these fabrics are made with chemicals, they pose no outgassing risks as a finished product, and they can significantly improve survival rates should a mattress be involved in a fire. At my company, Organic Mattresses, Inc., we manufacture organic mattresses with or without the liner depending upon the customer's preference.

Chapter   Seven

Beware, Greenwashers

"All that glitters is not green." —W.L. Bader

REMEMBER THE STORY of Rumpelstiltskin? The miller had a daughter who was reputed to be able to spin straw into gold. The rumor of her attributes was actually spread by her father to make himself appear more important, and he gave little thought to the consequences. Of course, when the king insisted that she prove this talent, the deception was obvious.

Unfortunately, in a world awash in greenwashing, the deception is not always as clear. But in similar fashion, greenwashers try to paint their companies and their products with attributes they don't possess. In politics they call it "spin." It's like Halloween where everyone comes to your door wearing a green costume and you have to try to figure out who's who.

Evidence is piling up about just how pervasive greenwashing is in the U.S. marketplace. In 2007, a research company went into a well-known big-box retailer and evaluated the environmental and "green" marketing claims of over 1,000 products. Only one lived up to its claims. That means that 999 of the products used deceptive advertising—false statements, self-made logos and "eco" branding, phony organizations, and membership emblems intended to infer that an organization has sanctioned a product, all designed to mislead consumers.

In 2009, TerraChoice, an environmental marketing company, estimated that between 2007 and 2008 the number of "green" products offered to consumers increased by almost 80 percent. And in a recent article entitled "American Shoppers Misled by Greenwash, Congress Told," British website guardian.co.uk states that "More than 98 percent of supposedly natural and environmentally friendly products on U.S. supermarket shelves are making potentially false or misleading claims … and 22 percent of products making green claims bear an environmental badge that has no inherent meaning." (guardian.co.uk/world/2009/jun/21/green-environment-ecology-congress-us-supermarkets)

Greenwashing is simply whitewashing using a different color. It uses disinformation, incomplete information, and fraudulent information to communicate "green" advantages that don't exist.

Greenwashing is everywhere, and the mattress industry could be its poster child. Today's memory-foam, polyurethane, synthetic latex, and thermoplastic fabrics are in fact as "black" as oil even though they are being touted as "green." Such ingredients, which are built into almost all popular mattresses, come from barrels of crude, not plants.

A favorite method to claim green, natural, or organic advantages is to use one or two raw materials that actually are legitimate, then claim the product is "green." Yes, it's true, some manufacturers substitute plant-based materials for part of the polyurethane in their mattress cores and layers, and then call it "green." (Well, you could say the oil did come from plants way back when, but the chemical derivatives used to create the artificial raw materials used in mattresses today are anything but green.)

While substituting soy or castor-bean derivatives for some of the chemical-based material in their formulas is better than nothing, touting it as somehow "green" is like being a little bit pregnant. An honest way of presenting their accomplishment would be to list the percentages of both plant-based and oil-derived ingredients. Instead, we see products with banner headlines that stress the "green" attribute with no mention of the "black" or oil-derived components—greenwashing by omission.

It has become popular in the mattress industry to describe products using *shades* of green—green, greener, and greenest. The problem with this strategy is that "green" has no base definition.

What such companies are really saying is this mattress has some chemicals, this one has fewer, and this one has the least, but they're not giving you any information about what's actually outgassing from these mattresses. They put their best foot forward, and their back foot carries the toxic burden.

I can tell you something for sure: Even a few PBDEs in your mattress can mean quite a lot in your body. Even if some of the carcinogenic materials in the polyurethane core contain a bit of plant-based material.

If you're going to go green, go all the way.

I've seen trade organizations invent self-serving rating systems, complete with slick logos that have no on-site verifications, enforcement component, or year-to-year compliance procedures—"green" tags designed to serve the needs of their members. (The most outrageous example I've found was an organization with an impressive "green" name that had only one member— the business that created it.)

Then you have the example of packaging designed to convey "green" images of blue skies and flowered meadows, hiding products inside that are full of toxic chemicals just like their competitive counterparts—pretty pictures, vague claims, and no proof.

Another technique is to make a donation or sponsor a "green" group, then capitalize on the inference that your company or products are green by association.

While there is a dire need for "green" product definitions and enforceable performance and ingredient standards, I suspect it will be easier for legislative bodies and committees to define greenwashing than to provide a concise definition of the word "green."

Bottom line: *Caveat emptor*—consumer beware.

Third-party Certifications Can Offer Consumers Proof that Products are Honestly Green

Reading labels can get boring fast, so relying on the logo of a legitimate certifying organization is an excellent way for consumers to find out who can really weave straw into gold.

While a recent study showed that consumers think the word "natural" is somehow regulated by government organizations, that is incorrect.

The only word that actually has legislative definition, enforcement provisions, and approved third-party designation by the United States Department of Agriculture (USDA) is the word "organic."

Certified organic food and beverage products are fairly well understood by most shoppers, but when the term is used on textile products it gets a little trickier to understand who is claiming what.

Every industry, product, or service has an applicable list of credible third-party organizations that validate standards. Standards such as the Global Organic Textile Standard (GOTS) can be verified by any number of independent organizations. Programs such as Oeko-Tex® and GREEN-GUARD® are important verifiers of information on specific harmful substances.

GREENGUARD is a highly respected U.S. organization that has the capacity to test finished consumer textile products, including mattresses, for the presence of harmful VOCs.

Organic Mattresses, Inc. and Lifekind® have been using GREENGUARD to test for toxic substances in their mattresses since 2006, and offer GREEN-GUARD written certification for their products.

Independent Websites Can Help or Mislead

The web is great, but it's important to remember that seldom is the information it contains verified for accuracy. However, there are some organizations that can give impartial advice.

For instance, www.betterworldshopper.org uses five criteria—the environment, animal protection, human rights, social justice, and community involvement—to evaluate over 1,000 major companies.

Be wary of websites that offer product reviews or rankings that don't provide open identification of site ownership or phone and address information so you can contact them to ask about the criteria they use and impartiality. More than likely it is a sham site that was designed to list the site designers' product first and then list leading competitors lower than themselves—greenwashing in a subtle form, or you could even call it green*scamming*.

From a practical standpoint, the web is like the Wild West in which there's no sheriff. For instance, a google search for "organic mattress" will produce over 400,000 results. Hundreds of these sites claim to make their products in an "organic mattress factory," but what exactly does that mean?

Using Organic Mattresses, Inc. as an example, here is how they justify the use of the term "organic mattress factory." First, their facility was built expressly for the manufacture of only organic products, and there is no chance of any cross contamination because they make no hybrid or synthetic products. Second, their facility is independently certified by a USDA-approved third-party organic certifying organization to the world-respected GOTS standard. Third, all their organic raw materials are lot-tracked and audited by an independent third-party certifier as well.

Who Protects Consumers From Greenwashing?

While every state has a Bureau of Consumer Protection to protect its citizens from fraudulent business practices and unfair competitive claims, section 5 of the Federal Trade Commission (FTC) Act authorizes the agency to intervene when trade misrepresentations occur in order to prevent consumer deception.

For example, in February 2010, the FTC sent warning letters to about 80 retailers, including Wal-Mart, Target, Kmart, Macy's, and Bed, Bath & Beyond, informing them that labeling rayon as bamboo is misleading and that claiming bamboo fabrics have environmental and antimicrobial advantages and are biodegradable in a landfill may also lead to civil suits. The FTC publishes a publication called *The Green Guides* specifically to help organizations understand the boundaries between marketing and fraud. A complete list of the companies can be found at www.ftc.gov/bamboo.

But it's not just about bamboo fabrics. Greenwashing has also been prevalent regarding hemp fabrics. Often the focus is on the fact that hemp grows in an environmentally friendly manner without evaluating the chemicals used to soften it enough to be suitable for clothing or bed linens. Most consumers are also unaware that much hemp comes from China and can be dyed without evaluating toxicity to workers or consumers.

Cotton is another textile that, while it may be grown organically, represents an extremely small percentage of worldwide cotton production. It is the number-one crop treated with chemical fertilizers and other applications.

Consumers are increasingly turning to the court system for redress. Class-action suits are pending against S. C. Johnson's "Greenlist" label, Tide, Ajax, and Windex, as well as hybrid automobile manufacturers and residential home builders.

In addition to FTC oversight, false advertising claims can also be pursued by the attorney general of your state under parallel state legislation. Competitors can even sue other businesses under Section 43(a) of the Lanham Act, 15 U.S.C. 1125(a) and state unfair competition or unfair business practices.

Have you been greenwashed? A concise list of the "Seven Sins of Greenwashing" can be found at www.sinsofgreenwashing.org/findings/the-seven-sins/. If you feel you've been greenwashed, a complaint can be filed at www.gov/ftc/complaint.shtm or by calling 1-877-382-4357.

Chapter Eight

How to Shop for an Organic Mattress

Ask anyone, "What are the most important criteria in shopping for a mattress?" and the instant reply is most frequently, "Comfort." A high level of comfort can be achieved by choosing the right materials in the manufacture of an organic mattress. As a bonus, organic mattresses are safer, too.

It always amazes me that people shop for a mattress with preconceptions of firmness. It is as if they were raised with a concept that firm mattresses are best, and soft mattresses are bad because they offer no support. In fact, either a firm, medium, or soft mattress may work for any given sleeper depending on his or her age, sleeping position, health conditions, and surface-softness preference.

Mattresses and Age

Age is a factor few people take into consideration when buying a mattress. As we get older, our circulation is not as vibrant, and our veins and arteries have less elasticity. This means that a firm mattress, which may have been comfortable when one was younger, may now create pressure points that reduce circulation to areas of the body, creating muscle pain and soreness. This is often the reason sleepers have to change position frequently or wake up in the morning feeling like they have been hit by a truck. These "pressure points" (or lack of circulation) are what cause bedsores when older people spend long periods of time in bed. Children, on the other hand, can fall asleep on a wood floor and wake up without any pain, because their circulatory systems are so young and healthy.

Mattresses and Sleeping Position

Sleeping position can dramatically influence which mattress is best for you. It indicates which parts of the body are in direct contact with the mattress surface, which in turn determines where pressure is being placed against the sleeper's body. People who are predominantly stomach or back sleepers can usually sleep comfortably on a firm—or even a very firm—mattress because their weight is being distributed evenly over the entire surface. On the other hand, side sleepers—the majority of Americans, research shows—usually require a softer mattress because they are placing the weight of their hips and shoulders directly against the mattress surface. In such cases, if the mattress is too firm it will not conform to the sleeper's weight, creating a pressure zone that cuts off circulation to that area, creating pain and discomfort. For these reasons, side sleepers are usually more comfortable on a soft, medium, or medium-firm mattress, often with a pillow top, which will minimize pressure points.

Orthopedic doctors frequently recommend a firm mattress for stomach and back sleepers because it will not allow the spine to sink into the surface, which can create unnatural angles and pressure on the spinal column. Stomach and back sleepers usually need a firmer mattress than do side sleepers to prevent this spinal distortion, which is usually manifested as morning pain. In fact, the most frequent symptom of stomach and back sleepers who sleep on mattresses that have lost their support or are too soft is waking up with lower back pain. People who sleep in these positions need a mattress that offers enough support, yet is soft enough to fill in the gaps in the contour of the back.

Mattress Surface Softness

Modern commercial mattresses seem to be designed to provide mattress shoppers with a surface that produces an instant soft gratification—and they certainly can feel good if you go mattress shopping directly after work. Pillow-top mattresses are ideal if the sleeper wants to be surrounded by a soft layer of comfort. However, if you have purchased the correct mattress firmness, you should not need a pillow top for functional support. Surveys of mattress shoppers have indicated that the average time a shopper lies on a mattress in a retail showroom is less than two minutes, so pillow tops can be a great instant selling tool. If you like that soft, "nesting" feeling and don't mind the body impressions that will be created over time, then by all means you should get one.

Mattresses and Health Conditions

With the exception of therapeutic beds designed to treat burn victims, I do not believe that any mattress or mattress pad has any healing powers. However, certain mattresses are more suitable than others for various health conditions.

For instance, a natural rubber mattress with a wool pillow-top layer over a ribbed or egg-crate-style top layer works well for sleepers who spend long periods of time in bed, because such a mattress increases air circulation beneath the body and reduces pressure-point contact. This kind of surface is often beneficial for people suffering from fibromyalgia. Likewise, a very firm mattress may be indicated for specific spinal injuries or following spinal surgery. Similarly, electric beds that allow the head of the mattress to elevate can help conditions such as asthma, acid reflux disorder, heart failure, and chronic lung disease. Natural rubber organic mattresses are an ideal choice for sleepers seeking an organic mattress for an electric bed.

Organic Mattress Materials Are Environmentally Friendly

Organic mattresses made with certified organic cotton, organic wool, and 100 percent natural rubber latex provide a safe and comfortable sleeping environment without the use of synthetic products made from nonrenewable resources that risk environmental damage. The life of such organic mattresses is easily 20 years or more, and at the end of their life cycle they are 100 percent biodegradable.

Certified Organic Cotton

Organic cotton is a natural, earth-friendly, renewable resource. When selecting an organic mattress, make certain that all paddings and cover fabrics are made with *certified* organic cotton. Do not accept substitutes such as "green cotton," "unbleached and undyed cotton," or "100 percent natural cotton." These descriptions are potentially misleading marketing expressions that describe cotton grown with pesticides and other chemicals.

Organically grown cotton is certified by independent third parties, and some state agencies, to ensure that no synthetic substances were used in its cultivation and harvesting. All certified organic cotton is guaranteed by the certifying entity to be grown without the use of synthetic pesticides, herbicides, defoliants, or fertilizers. No synthetic chemicals are used to strip the leaves in preparation for harvest or during the manufacturing process.

Only cotton grown on land free of chemicals for three years can be certified as organic, although cotton grown on fields free of chemicals for less than three years can be certified as "transitional organic." The stamp of approval from an independent third-party agency ensures that organic standards have been followed and that social rights have been observed in cotton production.

Commercially grown cotton (non-certified) is potentially harmful to human health, as well as to the local and global environment. During the past decades, environmental organizations have focused on the cotton industry as one of agriculture's most environmentally destructive entities. Research has found that growing and harvesting a single pound of cotton fiber uses one-third of a pound of chemicals. This in turn takes an enormous toll on the air, water, and soil, not to mention the health of people living and working in "cotton country." When choosing an organic mattress, pillow top, or top-of-bed linens, you are making a choice to support the elimination of these chemicals.

Most people are not aware that certified organic cotton grows naturally in shades of brown and green. Certified color-grown cotton fabrics in subtle hues of both these colors are achieved without dyes.

An interesting aside is that cotton is a food, as well as a fiber. Seeds and fibers are fed to cattle, and cottonseed oil is a main ingredient in processed foods. Since the federal government classifies cotton as a fiber, not a food source, farmers can use heavy amounts of toxic chemicals to produce it.

Pure Organic Wool

Wool is the perfect fiber for mattress padding. It is a safe, natural, mildew-resistant fiber that science cannot imitate for its breathability, versatility, practicality, and fire retardancy. Wool is nature's ideal insulator, keeping one cooler in summer and warmer in winter. Commonly chosen for its warmth, its insulating properties work both ways, making it an ideal material for beds and bedding. (The Bedouin people of the Sahara Desert actually wear wool to keep the heat *out*.)

Natural wool can absorb one-third of its weight in moisture before feeling wet, yet water evaporates quickly from it due to the air channels between the fibers. Since humans produce about a pint of water vapor during an eight-hour sleep cycle, wool provides an excellent "wicking" action that keeps sleepers' skin dry instead of wet and clammy.

Wool is also a renewable resource when harvested without slaughtering the sheep. Organic wool is produced on farms where sheep are fed and cared for without the use of toxic chemicals. Sheep raised organically do not receive routine chemical treatments such as drenching, dipping for parasites, fly dressing, antibiotics, growth hormones, or vaccines, nor do they graze on pastures that have been sprayed with herbicides. Genetically engineered or modified feed is prohibited. Rather, sheep raised organically graze only on organic fields and are fed organic stock food that helps them build healthy immune systems naturally. They are bred for resistance to parasites without using genetically engineered techniques.

The wool used in an organic mattress must adhere to meticulous inspection (i.e., for pests, dirt, and fiber length), and is raised using hygiene practices that eliminate the need for chemical treatments such as carbonizing. Only hot water and biodegradable soap are used to wash the wool, and no sulfuric-acid solution is used to dissolve vegetable materials. The wool is then hand selected for "carding" (the process of combing wool into batts used for padding and bedding).

Not only is wool the most breathable and insulating natural fiber on the planet, but if an organic mattress is constructed properly, the wool it contains will allow the product to meet federal flammability standards without the addition of toxic fire retardants.

Natural Rubber Latex

Natural rubber latex is an excellent core material for mattresses. It is resistant to mold, mildew, and bacteria, and dust mites will not live in a natural rubber environment. Natural rubber mattresses provide excellent support in any sleeping position, and instantly conform to any body shape. Natural rubber has been proven by pressure-sensing tests to produce fewer pressure points than do memory-foam mattresses.

We have come to view "latex" as a synthetic product, but in fact natural rubber latex is a renewable resource, as opposed to synthetic latex, which is made from petroleum derivatives. Pure natural rubber latex comes from the "milk," or latex, of the rubber tree (*Hevea brasiliensis*). Natural rubber latex is collected in much the same way that farmers tap maple trees for sap. Unlike sap that runs deep inside the tree, natural rubber latex milk runs in the tree's latex ducts, the layer immediately outside the cambium. Farmers take great care during harvesting to keep the tree healthy, since damage to the cambium stops tree growth (and thus future latex production).

When choosing a natural rubber or "latex" mattress, be suspicious of information found on the label. Sometimes the problem is a lack of information, since no law requires manufacturers to disclose the percentage of natural latex sap used in their latex formulation (if they are using any at all).

You may also see labels that say "100 percent Talalay rubber" that may actually be made with 100 percent synthetic chemicals (styrene-butadiene, or artificial rubber) and a different manufacturing process than Talalay. Such a product may be made from synthetic rubber blended with polyurethane or natural latex sap.

For instance, at the time of this writing, there is a major supplier of natural latex mattress cores claiming that their latex cores are USDA certified organic, but no such final-product certification for latex mattress cores currently exists through the USDA or any other agency or certifier in the United States.

As for comfort, natural rubber mattresses are great for light sleepers because they absorb approximately 85 percent of normal sleeping movements. With a natural rubber mattress, you will hardly be aware of your partner getting up or turning over in bed. Natural rubber is also the most durable and elastic material available. Its elastic properties give natural rubber mattresses the ability to retain their shape and original firmness for many years. They also offer excellent heat and moisture regulation, air circulation, and a metal-free sleeping environment. Natural rubber latex mattresses have by far the largest share of the organic mattress market.

Top-of-Bed Products

A combination of organically grown cotton and wool offers superior materials for the pillow top and bedding you will want to use on your organic mattress. These products will further promote a safe and comfortable sleeping environment. Mattress pads, dust-mite barrier covers, pillows, sheets, blankets, and comforters are all available as certified organic items.

Avoid putting a polyester mattress pad on an organic mattress. Such a product will introduce chemicals into your bed environment, and it will insert a barrier between you and the wonderful attributes provided by the wool in your mattress. Organic pillows are made with the same materials used in an organic mattress: wool, cotton, and/or natural rubber latex. Wool comforters offer lightweight comfort with the insulating qualities discussed above under Pure Organic Wool. Also, European studies have determined that a sleeper's heart rate, as well as humidity next to the skin, is lower under a wool comforter than under a down or synthetic-filled comforter. Sheets made with organic cotton fabric are soft, comfortable, and durable. (When choosing sheets, avoid those that have been dyed. Even "low-impact" dyes use chemicals in their processes.)

Where Can You Buy an Organic Mattress?

Organic manufacturers use all of the traditional marketing channels in their sales strategies. They sell directly to the consumer, through retailers, and on websites. The number of brick-and-mortar furniture and bedding stores that offer organic mattresses, while limited, is growing rapidly. Enter the search term "organic mattress" into your web browser and you will find roughly a million pages of information. Although there are many outlets through which consumers can purchase an organic mattress, there are actually only a handful of true manufacturers that produce organic mattresses and bedding. In addition, there is another type of manufacturer (an assembler) that purchases finished mattress components from a number of sources, and then assembles them into the final product. A true manufacturer, as opposed to an assembler, completes the entire manufacturing process—including quilting, cutting, and sewing—on their premises. Some manufacturers also produce conventional or "chemical" products in the same facility, which runs the risk of chemical cross-contamination from non-organic materials or products. This can be even more of a concern for the assembler type of manufacturer that buys its components from a number of outside sources.

Not only can organic mattresses be made in different types of production environments, but they can also be made with organic materials from a variety of sources. Furthermore, it is possible to go into a mainstream mattress store seeking an organic mattress and be misled by a misinformed salesperson. For example, I recently shopped a major mattress chain store, and patiently listened while the salesperson tried to convince me that a particular mattress was organic. At the conclusion of the presentation, I walked to the head of the bed and read to him the materials listed on the "law label" attached to the product. When I pointed out that polyurethane (which comprised 69 percent of the mattress) was not organic, but rather a chemical, he said he was unaware of that fact. Also, some salespeople use the words "natural" and "organic" as if they are one and the same, and the word "certified" seldom enters the conversation.

When Shopping for an Organic Mattress, Look For These Certifications

Taking a page from the organic food industry, organic products need three components to be recognized by the USDA/National Organic Program (NOP): certified raw materials, a certified manufacturing process, and assurances that the final product has been tested for contamination.

As previously mentioned, currently no USDA/NOP certification exists for mattresses. Nevertheless, third-party certification of the raw materials and manufacturing process, along with product testing, can still be done to assure consumers that the product they are purchasing is not just being assembled in someone's garage with a sewing machine and a tape-edge binder—or put together in an environment that primarily produces "chemical" mattresses.

Certified organic materials are not hard to find. Any number of suppliers offer them with a variety of valid certifications, but how does one verify that just because a company has a certificate posted on the web or in their literature that this is in fact what was used to make their mattress? This is where third-party certification of the factory becomes critical. For example, the Organic Mattresses, Inc. (OMI) facility has been third-party independently certified to the world-recognized Global Organic Textile Standard (GOTS). The certifying organization sends out inspectors who check not only the facility, but also the certifications, and audits the factory to make sure that end products are tracked back to the certified organic materials that are claimed to have been used in the products.

Finally, OMI-finished products are tested by GREENGUARD®, another independent third party, for VOC emissions. Here is where it gets a little complicated. What some manufacturers are doing to get around expensive VOC product testing is to accept the results of their supplier, who has submitted its products to a laboratory that identifies whether or not specific chemicals are being emitted. The supplier uses a laboratory that tests for specific chemicals, and then uses that test to say that no VOCs have been detected. Clever, but it doesn't give the consumer any information as to what is actually coming out of a mattress. This is similar to a company saying that its raw materials are GOTS certified, therefore their mattresses are GOTS certified. Unfortunately, since contamination and substitution of raw materials can occur at any time during the manufacturing process, this is one of those times when the sum of the parts may not equal the whole.

Organic mattress shoppers also need to be aware that there is no legal requirement that any mattress manufacturer inform consumers if it is using chemicals in its latex blend or foam cores that enable them to comply with state and federal flammability laws.

Flammability standards can be met without chemicals. OMI proved to the Consumer Products Safety Commission, when they were audited in March 2008 and during California state audits in 2006, 2007 and 2009, that flammability requirements can be met by using only organic wool without any chemical fire retardants. Its brand, organicpedic®, can be found in organically conscious retail mattress stores throughout the United States and Canada (www.organicpedicbyOMI.com).

The Smart Shopper's Guide to Mattress Brands

In 2010, the Green Patriot Working Group and *The Doctors' Prescription for Healthy Living*, two consumer organizations and media companies I recommend, did an in-depth survey of many major mattress companies that are offering what they term "green" mattress and bedding products. Were they really green? Which were the best? These are the questions their reporters asked via phone and questionnaire.

The results showed exactly what I have seen: that indeed there are various shades of green, but that many companies actually use a substantial amount of toxic oil-based materials.

In the chart below, overall score is based mainly on third-party inspection of production facilities and testing for contaminants, along with raw-material certifications. It takes more than just ingredients to label a product organic. A product can't claim to be an organic product without third-party inspection of the production facilities and testing for contaminants.

For further comparison, please check the tables below regarding processes, testing, and certifications.

Organic Mattress Shopping Checklist

(provided by the Green Patriot Working Group and Healthy Living *magazine)*

Production Facility & Finished Product Certifications

Rank	Brand/Model	Location	100% organic production	GOTS-certified facility	Final product tested for VOC emissions	Final product tested for flammability
1	OMI/OrganicPedic	USA	✔	✔	✔	✔
2	Lifekind	USA	✔	✔	✔	✔
3	Natura World—Organic Series	Canada				✔
4	Vivetique Organic Cotton	USA				✔
5	WJS Southard—1915 Collection	USA				✔
6	White Lotus 100% Organic	USA				✔
7	Land & Sky Organic Mattress	USA				✔
8	Simmons—Organic Series	USA				N/A

Raw Material Certifications*

Rank	Brand/Model	Cotton	Ticking	Thread, Canvas	Barrier Cover	Wool	Water-based Adhesive	3rd-Party Verification? Yes. GOTS-Certified	No. Claimed Only by Manufacturer
1	OMI/OrganicPedic	✔	✔	✔	✔	✔	✔	✔	
2	Lifekind	✔	✔	✔	✔	✔	✔	✔	
3	Natura World—Organic Series	✔	✔		✔	✔	✔		✔
4	Vivetique Organic Cotton	✔	✔		✔	✔	✔		✔
5	WJS Southard—1915 Collection	✔	✔			✔	✔		✔
6	White Lotus 100% Organic	✔							✔
7	Land & Sky Organic Mattress	✔	✔		✔	✔			✔
8	Simmons—Natural Care								✔

continued

Materials Used*

Rank	Brand/Model	Contains polyurethane foam	Made with 100% natural latex	Contains synthetic latex	Fire resistance	What's inside?	What's outside?
1	OMI/OrganicPedic		✔		Eco-Wool™	100% natural latex	Eco-Wool, organic cotton
2	Lifekind		✔		Naturally Safer® Pure Wool	Talalay natural rubber	Organic cotton, Naturally Safer® Pure Wool
3	Natura World— Organic Series		✔		All-natural wool & fabric barrier	100% natural latex core	Organic wool & cotton
4	Vivetique Organic Cotton		✔		Naturally fire resistant	Organic cotton, PureGrow wool, natural latex	Organic cotton ticking
5	WJS Southard— 1915 Collection		✔		Organic & eco-friendly wool	Horsehair, organic wool, organic cotton, flax, Talalay latex	Organic cotton
6	White Lotus 100% Organic		✔		None listed	Organic cotton, natural latex	Organic cotton
7	Land & Sky Organic Mattress		✔		Natural wool fill	Organic cotton, organic wool, natural latex, untreated & unstained wood	Organic cotton (unbleached & not dyed), natural latex
8	Simmons— Natural Care	N/A	65%	N/A	None listed	Natural latex, soy	None listed

* Only OMI and Lifekind have submitted to third-party facility verification (GOTS) of their products and facility. We cannot verify the other manufacturers' claims and cannot guarantee that the representations they have made have been verified by any third party.

Buying an organic mattress? How do other mattresses compare? There are so many ways nowadays that companies convey their message with different degrees of truthfulness. "The whole truth and nothing but the truth" should be the standard, but there are so many areas of concern that it is difficult to make your decision without an objective helper.

Unless you know the questions to ask you won't know how organic or nontoxic your mattress really is. At this time, there are no federal standards for organic mattresses.

Remember there are three parts to buying an organic mattress: (1) Raw Materials; (2) Production Facility; and (3) Final Product Testing. And prepare to be lied to.

Companies claiming to be manufacturers or using organic ingredients often have certifications that are outdated by years.

However, our reporters have put together this checklist to make sure you are purchasing the highest-quality, safest, and most comfortable organic mattress. Use this checklist when comparing "green" mattresses.

Note that in this checklist we have listed typical and often the best third-party certifying organizations for each component of a mattress. While a company might not have the exact same certifications as listed below, they should demonstrate the same level of integrity:

Yes No

RAW MATERIALS CERTIFICATIONS

☐ ☐ Organic Cotton Fill *National Organic Program (NOP) Certified*

☐ ☐ Certified Organic *Ticking Global Organic Textile Standard (GOTS)*

☐ ☐ Latex *Oeko-Tex Environment-Safe Certified*

☐ ☐ Thread, Flannel and Canvas *GOTS-Certified Organic*

☐ ☐ Sateen and Barrier Cover *NOP Certified Organic*

☐ ☐ Wool *USDA Animal-Welfare Certified*

☐ ☐ Water-Based Adhesive *GREENGUARD Certified*

☐ ☐ Raw Materials *American Sourced*

PRODUCTION FACILITY AND PROCESSES

☐ ☐ Dedicated 100% U.S. Organic Mattress Eco-Factory™

☐ ☐ Sanitized Raw Materials (non-pesticide)

☐ ☐ GOTS-Certified Factory

FINISHED PRODUCT CERTIFICATION AND TESTING

☐ ☐ Certified by GREENGUARD for low VOC emissions

☐ ☐ Consumer Products Safety Commission (CPSC) Flammability Tested and Approved

For more information about this independent consumer project, visit www.safebedroom.com and www.greenpatriot.us.

Final Thoughts

"The woods are lovely, dark and deep.
But I have promises to keep,
and miles to go before I sleep."
—Robert Frost, 1923
(in *Stopping By Woods On A Snowy Evening*)

In 1994, Vice President Al Gore wrote in his introduction for a new edition of Rachel Carson's book *Silent Spring* that "the power of an idea can be far greater than the power of politicians." This book was intended to contribute "power" to the idea that humans have a right to live in an uncontaminated environment.

While I have focused my comments on the bedroom—and more specifically mattresses—because I believe this is the simplest way to avoid chemicals in a major part of your life (sleeping), we cannot lose sight of the larger issue. Politicians have the power to protect us from toxic consumer products and environmental contaminants. But this will only happen if we demand it.

Bed Bugs and Dust Mites: Which One Bites?

D<small>UST MITES EAT DEAD SKIN CELLS</small>; bed bugs eat you (although they will also feast on pets in a pinch). Good News: Neither one is a carrier of disease.

Dust mites are an unavoidable side effect of dust. Bed bugs travel into the home on clothing, used furniture, mattresses, or any fabric that has come into contact with them. Dust mites are microscopic (500 could live in a single gram of dust). Bed bugs can be seen with the naked eye (adults are about a quarter of an inch long and flat)—but good luck finding them.

Both live within mattresses and upholstered furniture, but while dust mites have a definite preference for the constant-humidity habitats found within furniture and mattresses, bed bugs are not as fussy and have been known to live within walls during the day, coming out at night to feed.

The medical community has recognized for some time that exposure to dust-mite allergens is one of the primary triggers of asthmatic reactions. Dust mites can also cause perennial allergic rhinitis. These symptoms occur because the body's immune system cannot cope with the offending allergens. It reacts by producing histamines, which in turn create the swelling and mucus production we often associate with hay fever or colds. Other allergic-rhinitis symptoms can include headache; dark circles under the eyes; sinus pressure; red, watery eyes; itchy throat, eyes, and ears; and sneezing. Your level of sensitivity to dust-mite allergens can easily be determined by your physician doing a simple skin-prick test or a RAST blood test.

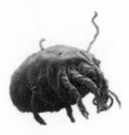

Dust mites love comforters and pillows. If you ever needed a reason to buy a new pillow, about 10 percent of the weight of a two-year-old pillow is actually dust-mite droppings (excrement). With one notable exception: dust mites do not like natural latex pillows and mattresses. This is because the holes in the latex serve as ventilation, keeping the humidity level lower than the mites prefer. Furthermore, natural rubber mattresses usually lack sufficient quantities of padding to ensure the constant temperature and humidity they require. In comparison, dust mites can make a home within mattresses made from polyurethane formulas, which is why many foam formulas specifically add chemicals to make the material more dust-mite resistant.

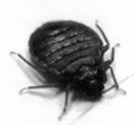

Bed bugs can come from any number of sources: visitors, hotel rooms, animals, and especially used furniture and clothing. While neither dust mites nor bed bugs carry disease, bed-bug bites are itchy, and infection can occur from scratching. The bites look like a small red or whitish raised area, and you will usually discover them in the morning, since they are nocturnal feeders.

Bed-bug trails are not hard to spot on a mattress. They leave behind traces of blood, feces, eggs, skin cells, and even their dead. Not information you probably want to hear, but there are solutions.

Controlling Dust Mites and Bed Bugs

Barrier covers work to keep the critters from coming out of your mattress or pillows (or from getting into them in the first place), and can be an effective solution. Look for barrier covers made from certified organic cotton to avoid the chemical offgassing that can occur from covers made from PVC vinyl or other forms of plastic. (Keep in mind that if bed bugs are living elsewhere in the room, such as in walls or in a chair adjacent to your bed, they are going to find you when they go out for their "evening stroll" no matter how well your mattress is protected.)

I am not a particular fan of trying to reduce dust mites and bed-bug infestations with air-purification systems. First of all, the bugs and mites don't fly, so airborne solutions don't really work. In my opinion, even air filters with high-energy particle arresting (HEPA) filters capable of trapping very small particles are not effective.

A number of aerosol sprays, insecticides, and bed-bug traps are available. (I favor the traps, since the chemicals they contain have less of a chance of entering your skin or lungs.) Treating just one room will usually not rid you of these pests, and more and more of these bug populations are showing up with resistance to insecticides, making control increasingly difficult.

One caveat: Seldom do these products have a complete list of their ingredients, which makes assessing the chemical risks from the treatment challenging. This is especially important to understand relative to young children and pets.

About the Pesticides NOT in Certified Organic Cotton

THE PESTICIDES WE USE to control weeds and insects in and around our homes can be significant health hazards. Exposure to certain pesticides is associated with health problems ranging from skin rashes to nervous-system disorders and cancer. Children are at the greatest risk of harm because of their hand-to-mouth habits and still-developing nervous systems; also, the places where they play are often the types of areas that are treated with pesticides. In recent years, a number of the most dangerous pesticides have been pulled off the market, thanks to pressure from environmental groups. But that doesn't make the aging supplies in your garage any safer.

According to the EPA, 75 percent of households in the U.S. used at least one pesticide product indoors during the past year. And a recent study sponsored by the EPA found that the number and concentration of pesticides detected in indoor air is generally greater than that found in outdoor air. People are exposed to pesticides by inhaling them or accidentally coming into contact with them. Many people bring pesticides into their homes in the form of insecticides, fungicides, and disinfectants. These products are sold as sprays, liquids, sticks, powders, crystals, balls, and foggers. Pesticides can also be tracked into a home on the soles of shoes or on pets' feet, or they can waft in from the outdoor air. A study published in *Archives of Environmental Contamination and Toxicology* found that pesticides can be detected in indoor air even when there has not been pesticide use on the property.

In 2002, the American Association of Poison Control Centers reported that over 96,000 people were involved in common household pesticide poisonings or exposures. More than 50,000 of these cases involved children under the age of six.

It is important to remember that pesticides are products that are intended to kill something, whether it's an ant or a fungus. These products can be dangerous if they are allowed to accumulate inside the home.

There are safer alternatives to chemical pesticides. Keeping your home and its surroundings clean and well maintained will go a long way toward discouraging pests and other problems. Remove your shoes when you enter your house, as they can track in harmful pesticides, lead, cadmium, and other chemicals. Keeping a floor mat at your door for people to wipe their feet on when they enter will help as well. It is also a good idea to vacuum carpets and floors regularly. Children playing on carpeting may be exposed to pesticides lodged in the carpet at higher levels than outside, since pesticides break down less readily indoors than they do outdoors in the sunlight.

Avoid pesticides that contain organophosphates, which include acephate, dichlorvos, dimethoate, disulfoton, malathion, naled, phosmet, tetrachlorvinphos, and trichlorfon. Carbamates, which include the pesticides carbaryl (Sevin) and propoxur (Baygon), are another class of chemicals that should be avoided. The dangerous pesticide diazinon was banned at the end of 2004, but may still be found in older bottles of herbicides in your home or on store shelves. Likewise, the manufacture of chlorpyrifos (sold as Dursban or Lorsban) was halted as of 2000, but stores were still allowed to sell existing stocks, which were considerable. If you find unsafe pesticides in your home, don't flush them down a toilet or pour them down a drain. These chemicals don't belong in your home or in our water supply. Instead, call your local public-works department to find out how to dispose of unsafe pesticides. Also, lobby your local government not to use unnecessary or unsafe pesticides in parks, schools, and other public places.

The primary agency created to protect America's health from toxic exposures is the Department of Health and Human Services, Agency for Toxic Substances and Disease Registry, 1825 Century Blvd., Atlanta, GA 30345, Public Inquiries: 888-422-8737. Other important sources and publications are listed below:

The Environmental Protection Agency (EPA)
Public Information Center
401 M Street, SW PM-20460
Recommended Publications: *Carpet and Indoor Air Quality, Biological Pollutants in Your Home, An Update on Formaldehyde, Citizen's Guide to Pesticides*

The Consumer Product Safety Commission
Chemical Hazards Program
5401 Westbard Avenue, Room 419
Bethesda, MD 20207
Recommended Publication: *The Inside Story: A Guide to Indoor Air Quality*

The National Academy of Science
500 Fifth Street, N.W.
Washington, D.C. 20001
Recommended Publication: *Human Bio-monitoring for Environmental Chemicals* (2006)

Consumer Information Center
Department 620-Y
Pueblo, CO 81009
Recommended Publication: *Indoor Air Quality and New Carpet*

The American Lung Association
1740 Broadway
New York, NY 10019
Recommended Publication: *Home Control of Allergies and Asthma*

Suggested Reading

Synthetic Planet: Chemicals, Politics and the Hazards of Modern Life **by Monica Casper, Rutledge, 2003**

An excellent explanation of the politics surrounding industrial chemicals.

Dying from Dioxin—A Citizen's Guide to Reclaiming Our Health and Rebuilding Democracy **by Lois Marie Gibbs, South End Press, 1995**

Explains how dioxin is everywhere, and goes on to detail this serious threat to our health.

Toxic Deception: How the Chemical Industry Manipulates Science, Bends the Law and Endangers Your Health **by Dan Fagin, Marianne Lavelle, and the Center for Public Integrity, Common Courage Press, 1999**

An investigative reporter's views of the chemical industry, pointing out many interesting facts and relationships, i.e., almost 50 percent of the top officials who left their employment with the Environmental Protection Agency (EPA) in the past 15 years now work for chemical companies.

Chemical Exposures: Low Levels and High Stakes **by Nicholas Ashford and Claudia Miller, Van Nostrand Reinhold, 1998**

A good exploration into the concept of individual sensitivity to low-level chemical exposures.

Our Toxic World: A Wake Up Call **by Dr. Doris Rapp, MD, Environmental Research Foundation, 2003**

Discusses how chemicals surrounding us affect not only our physical health but also our behaviors, and are the cause of a number of chronic illnesses.

Toxics A to Z: A Guide to Everyday Pollution Hazards **by John Harte, Cheryl Holdren, Richard Schneider and Christine Shirley, University of California Press, 1991**

A good place for the layperson to begin to understand the 100 most common toxins found in their surroundings.

The Consumer's Guide to Effective Environmental Choices: Practical Advice from the Union of Concerned Scientists **by Michael Brower and Warren Leon, Three Rivers Press, 1999**

A well-researched and down-to-earth guide for sensible environmental decision-making in your everyday life.

Chemical Deception: The Toxic Threat to Health and the Environment **by Marc Lappe, Sierra Club, 1992**

An early book that discredits many of the common statements surrounding the often-quoted claim by chemical-industry members that exposure to chemicals won't hurt you.

Seeds of Deception **by Jeffrey Smith, Chelsea Green Publishing, 2003**

The first book to disclose industry and government involvement with genetically modified foods.

Tired or Toxic: A Blueprint for Health by Sherry Rogers, Prestige Publications, 1990

An early work describing the sources of toxins and an individual's physical ability to deal with them.

Chemical Sensitivity by Sherry Rodgers, McGraw-Hill, 1998

An introduction to and explanation of Multiple Chemical Sensitivity (MCS) and body chemistry.

Creating A Healthy Household by Lynn Marie Bower, Healthy House Institute, 2000

This is an excellent book for those seeking specific product sources and basic information on their home environment.

Homes That Heal by Athena Thompson, New Society Publishers, 2004

The author gives a Bau-biologist's perspective on how your home can contribute to many health problems, and recommends solutions.

Safe Shopper's Bible by David Steinman and Samuel S. Epstein, Macmillan, 1995

A great reference source and guide that provides valuable toxic insights into everyday household products, cosmetics and food.

The Invisible Disease by Gunni Nordström, John Hunt Publishers, 2004

Discusses the dangers of environmental illnesses caused by electromagnetic fields and chemical emissions.

Diet for a Poisoned Planet: The 21st Century Edition by David Steinman, Avalon, 2007

How to choose safe foods for you and your family.

Living Green by Greg Horn, Freedom Press, 2006

A practical guide to simple sustainability.

Safe Trip to Eden by David Steinman, Avalon, 2007

Ten steps to save planet Earth from the global warming meltdown.

A p p e n d i x   F o u r

Websites

Centers for Disease Control and Prevention:
National Report on Human Exposure to Environmental Chemicals
www.cdc.gov/exposurereport

ChemFinder Database
www.chemfinder.camsoft.com

Chemical Body Burden
www.chemicalbodyburden.org

Chem-Tox: A consumer bulletin board that reports problems associated
with chemicals in mattresses.
www.chem-tox.com/guest/guestbook.html

Collaborative on Health and the Environment
www.healthandenvironment.org

EnviroLink Library
www.envirolink.org

Environmental Defense Fund's Chemical Scoreboard
www.scorecard.org

Environmental Facts Warehouse
www.epa.gov/enviro/

Environmental and Occupational Health Science Institute
www.eohsi.rutgers.edu

Forest Guardians
www.fguardians.org

Greenpeace, USA
www.greenpeace.org

Guide to Less Toxic Products
www.lesstoxicguide.ca

Mattress Illness Bulletin Board
Maintained by Wayne Sinclair, M.D. and Richard Pressinger, M.Ed.
www.chem-tox.com/beds/frame-beds.htm

National Health Information Center:
Health Information Resource Database
www.health.gov/nhic

National Resources Defense Council
www.nrdc.org

National Resources Defense Council:
Toxic Chemicals and Health Information
www.nrdc.org/health

PANNA (Pesticide Action Network North America)
www.panna.org

Physicians for Social Responsibility
www.psr.org

Sierra Club
www.sierraclub.org

Silent Spring Institute
www.silentspring.org

Union of Concerned Scientists
www.ucsusa.org

U.S. Department of Labor Occupational Safety and Health
Administration Hazardous Material Information Website
www.osha.gov/SLTC/hazardouswaste/index.html

U.S. Environmental Protection Agency
www.epa.gov

U.S. Environmental Protection Agency: Household Waste and Ecosystems
www.epa.gov/epaoswer/non-hw/muncpl/hhw.htm

Washington Toxics Coalition
www.watoxics.org

References

Chapter 1

Committee on Energy and Commerce. H.R.5820, *Toxic Chemicals Safety Act* of 2010. 22 July, 2010

California Department of Toxic Substances Control. National Report on *Human Exposure to Environmental Chemicals*. Retrieved on 8/6/2010 from http://www.cdc.gov/exposurereport

Department of Toxic Substances Control. California Green Chemistry Initiative; Final Report. December 2008

Cook, Kenneth. "Oral testimony, as delivered before the Subcommittee on Commerce, Trade and Consumer Protection Committee on Energy and Commerce". July 29, 2010.

California Department of Toxic Substances Control. DTSC Databases. Retrieved on 8/12/10 from http://www.dtsc.ca.gov/

California Green Chemistry Initiative: Frequently Asked Questions. December 2008. Retrieved on 8/6/10 from dtsc.ca.gov/GreenChemistry

Lautenberg Press Office. *Lautenberg Introduces "Safe Chemicals Act" to Protect Americans from Toxic Chemicals.* April 15, 2010. Retrieved on 8/13/10 from http://lautenberg.senate.gov/newsroom/record.cfm?id=323863

Chapter 2

Agency for Toxic Substances and Disease Registry (ATSDR). "Boron." Atlanta, GA: US Department of Health and Human Services, Public Health Service. 1995.

Agency for Toxic Substances and Disease Registry (ATSDR). *Managing Hazardous Materials Incidents. Volume III—Medical Management Guidelines for Acute Chemical Exposures: Methylene Chloride.* Atlanta, GA: U.S. Department of Health and Human Services, Public Health Service. 2001.

Alliance for the Polyurethanes Industry (API). "Hyperreactivity and Other Health Effects of Diisocyamates: Guidelines for the Medical Professional." Technical Bulletin, Jan 2000, AX150.

The Boston Channel, "Is Your Mattress Making You Sick?" Retrieved on 12/01/2005 from http://www.thebostonchannel.com/health/1792452/detail.html.

Environmental Working Group. *Mother's Milk.* Washington DC. 2005.

Hawthorne, M. "DuPont hit with $10 million fine." *Chicago Tribune,* December 15, 2005.

Hooper, K. and McDonals, T. "The PBDEs: An Emerging Environmental Challenge and Another Reason for Breast-Milk Monitoring Programs," *Environmental Health Perspectives,* 2000; 108(5):387-392.

Nandan, S. Bijoy, "The Pollution of Retting Coconuts on the Southwest Coast of India." *International Journal of Environmental Studies,* 1997;66(6).

Trevillian, L.F., Ponsonby, A.L., Dwyer, T., Kemp, A., Cochrane, J., Lim, L.Y., and Carmichael, A. "Infant Sleeping Environment and Asthma at 7 Years: A Prospective Cohort Study." *American Journal of Public Health,* December 2005; 95(12).

U.S. Department of Agriculture. "Agricultural Chemical Usage, 2003 Field Crops Summary." *National Agricultural Statistics Service,* Ag Ch1 (04)a, May, 2004.

U.S. Environmental Protection Agency. "Perfluorooctanoic Acid (PFOA)." Retrieved on 12/27/2005 from http://www.epa.gov/opptintr/pfoa/ngstatus.htm.

World Resources Institute. "Polyurethane Foam Project." Retrieved on 08/01/2002 from www.wri.org/meb/sei/polyfoam.html.

Chapter 3

Anderson, R.C. and Anderson, J.H. "Respiratory Toxicity of Mattress Emissions in Mice." *Archives of Environmental Health,* 2000 Jan-Feb;55(1):38-43.

Keimling, S.U. and Bader, M.R. "Burning Issues: Fire and Price." Nitroil Performace Chemicals, Germany.

Keimling, S.U. and Klockemann, W. "Bridging the Gap by High Activity: Low Emission but High Ageing Resistance." Nitroil Performance Chemicals, Germany.

Scientific Instrument Services. "Identification Of Volatile Organic Compounds in a New Automobile," Retrieved on 12/01/2005 from http://www.sisweb.com/referenc/applnote/ app-36-a.htm.

Sleep Products Safety Council. "Assessment of Potential Health Risks Resulting from Chemical Emissions from New Bedding Sets." *Proceedings of the Polyurethane Foam Association*, May 16 & 17, 1996.

U.S Environmental Protection Agency. "Sources of Indoor Air Pollution— Organic Gases (Volatile Organic Compounds-VOCs)." Retrieved on 11/18/2005 from http://www.epa.gov/iaq/voc.html.

U.S. Environmental Protection Agency. "Sources of Indoor Air Pollution— Pesticides." Retrieved on 11/19/2005 from http://www.epa.gov/iaq/pesticid.html.

U.S. Environmental Protection Agency. "Toxicological Review of Naphthalene. Agency for Toxic Substances and Disease Registry's (ATSDR's) Toxicological Profile for Naphthalene."

Chapter 4

Agency for Toxic Substances and Disease Registry, "ToxFAQs™ for Trichloroethylene (TCE)." Retrieved on 12/29/2005 from http://www.atsdr.cdc.gov/tfacts19.html.

Anderson, I. "Volatile Organic Compounds." *New Scientist*, 18 September 1986.

Anderson, R. "Toxic emissions from carpets." *Journal of Nutritional and Environmental Medicine*, 1995; 5: 375-386.

The Carpet and Rug Institute. "Facts About the Carpet Industry." Retrieved on 11/17/2005 from http://www.carpetrug.org/ drill_down_2.cfm?page=10&sub=3&requesttimeout=350.

Giardino, N.J. and Andelman, J.B. "Characterization of the emissions of trichloroethylene, chloroform, and 1,2-dibromo-3-chloropropane in a full-size, experimental shower." *J Exposure Anal Environ Epidemiol*, 1996;6: 413-423.

International Agency for Research on Cancer. "Tetrachloroethelyene." *Monographs,1995*; 63:159.

McKinlay, A.F. and Repacholi, M.H. "More research is needed to determine the safety of static magnetic fields." *Prog Biophys Molec Biol*, 2005;87:173-174.

The National Institute of Environmental Health Science. "Dry Cleaners: Perchloroethylene." Retrieved on 12/10/2005 from http://www.niehs.nih.gov/external/faq/dryclean.htm.

Possick, Kare, *Why Are You Poisoning Your Family, A Consumer Alert Publication.* The National Institute of Occupational Safety and Health. USA. 1994.

U.S. Environmental Protection Agency, "Indoor Air Facts No. 4 (revised): Sick Building Syndrome (SBS)." Retrieved on 11/17/2005 from http://www.epa.gov/iaq/pubs/sbs.html.

Weisel, C.P. and Jo, W.-K. "Ingestion, inhalation, and dermal exposures to chloroform and trichloroethene from tap water." *Environ. Health Perspect,* 1996; 104:48-51.

Woo, Ching S., Barry, S.E., and Zaromb, S. "Detection and estimation of part-per-billion levels of formaldehyde using a portable high-throughput liquid absorption air sampler." *Environmental Science & Technology,* Jan 1, 1998; 32(1)8.

Chapter 5

European Commission. "Eco-Label." Retrieved on 01/02/2006 from http://europa.eu.int/ comm/environment/ecolabel/tools/faq_en.htm.

Chapter 6

Krasny, J., Parker, W., and Babrauskas, V. *Fire Behavior of Upholstered Furniture and Mattresses.* Williams Andrews Publishing/Noyles, New York, 2001.

Sing, H., Singh, S., and Sharma, T.P. "Fire Retardant Studies on Polyurethane Foams." Retrieved on 01/03/2006 from http://www.pu-india.org/pu-newsletter2.htm.

U.S. Senate Committee on Commerce, Science and Transportation. "Testimony Submitted for Record," David Orders, July 2004. Retrieved on 11/21/2006 from http://commerce.senate.gov/hearings/ testimony.cfm?id=1267&wit_id=3728.

Appendix 2

Lewis, R.G., Fortmann, R.C. and Camann, D.E. "Evaluation of Methods for Monitoring the Potential Exposure of Small Children to Pesticides in the Residential Environment." *Arch Environ Contamin Toxicol,* 1994; 26:37-46.

U.S. Environmental Protection Agency, Office of Research and Development *Nonoccupational Pesticide Exposure Study (NOPES) Final Report.* EPA 600/3-90/003; US Government Printing Office: Washington, DC, 1990.

Watson, et al. 2002 *Annual Report of the American Association of Poison Control Centers. American Association of Poison Control Centers,* Washington, DC. 2002.

Index

About the Author

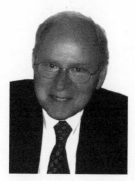

Having been chemically sensitive his whole life, Walt Bader is intimately aware of the chemical challenges that bombard us on a daily basis. His continual quest has been to find safer alternatives for the everyday products that he uses, and by so doing, to avoid the health risks associated with products that are routinely made with chemicals.

In 1995, he decided to share these products with others and co-founded Lifekind®, Inc., a national catalog company specializing in organic and Naturally Safer® product alternatives. Several years later, Walt and his partner created the first organic mattress Eco-Factory™—Organic Mattresses, Inc.—to produce their mattresses and other top-of-the-bed products.

For years Walt and his staff have been answering questions from consumers about the safety of their bedroom environments. Although he has sometimes wished he had been a chemistry major when dealing with the complexities of chemical composition, he realizes that his frustrations are typically what consumers feel as they try to assess the health risks posed by products made with unidentified and untested chemicals.

Walt did his undergraduate work in business and his graduate studies in law, and although they gave him the tools he needed to become a successful entrepreneur, he had to learn how to survive in this toxic world with a great deal of help from other individuals and publications.

Walt's first book, *Toxic Bedrooms: Your Guide to a Safe Night's Sleep*, was the first publication to let consumers know about the specific chemicals that outgas from conventional mattresses. *Sleep Safe in a Toxic World* expands his literary contribution with legislative updates, a new chapter on greenwashing, and information about raw materials and bedroom products that have come to market since *Toxic Bedrooms* was published in 2007.

Additional Titles Available
from Freedom Press

Extraordinary Healing by L. Stephen Coles, MD, PhD
Learn about the amazing discovery of destabilized DNA
by Dr. Mirko Beljanski and the health benefits of selective
plant molecules and RNA fragments.
$15.95

No More Allergies, Asthma, or Sinus Infections by Dr. Lon Jones
America's most famous country doctor shares a natural solution
for curing yourself of allergies, sinus problems and other
upper respiratory conditions.
$15.95

Living Green by Greg Horn
Practical advice and solutions for living lightly on the planet
while optimizing personal health.
$14.95

Patient Heal Thyself by Jordan Rubin
The story of Jordan Rubin's recovery from incurable illness
is one of the most dramatic natural healing stories ever told.
$19.95

Available at fine book retailers and health food stores

Also available at Amazon.com,
BarnesandNoble.com and Freedompressonline.com

Call 800.959.9797 for more information